A TIDE IN THE AFFAIRS OF MEDICINE

A TIDE IN THE AFFAIRS OF MEDICINE

National Health Insurance as the Augury of Professionalism

George M. Hall

WARREN H. GREEN
8356 Olive Blvd
St. Louis, MO 63132

Published by

Warren H. Green, Inc.
8356 Olive Boulevard
St. Louis, MO 63132 U.S.A.
314-991-1335
1-(800)-537-0655

ISBN 0-87527-536-2

First Printing 2004

For the selfless men and women
of the Salvation Army

TABLE OF CONTENTS

LIST OF ILLUSTRATIONS

LIST OF TABLES

Preface

THIS IS A revision to an earlier book written about ten years ago, under the title *Ethics and Economics of Health Care*. The text of the earlier book was more-or-less academic, as there was no chance at the time that national health insurance could become a reality. It was just food for thought. In the interim, matters changed and the publisher asked me to consider a revision.

At first, I thought this revision would consist primarily of updates to data and references. But a month-long survey of articles published in various newspapers and journals convinced me that the problems in health care finance were rapidly degenerating into an intolerable situation, where millions of Americans are uninsured or "under-insured" and HMOs and insurance companies are shifting life-or-death decisions from doctors to accountants.

This meant there was now a much stronger need for a national health insurance plan, and with it, a more forceful book—a complete rewrite with only one chapter surviving more-or-less intact. Moreover, advances made in computer and automation technology, will make the administrative implementation of any such plan more practical.

Hence this edition has a specific focus and presents the earlier proposed model in more detail, complete with various options and with the arguable advantages and disadvantages of each. Also, the discussions in the earlier book on ethical aspects have been integrated into the text.

As a personal note, my professional interests during the past decade turned to theology and history. The axes I am grinding remain in those fields, not in health care. Perhaps that makes my view of national health insurance more objective albeit at the price of personal commitment. On the other hand, if there is any one point that is emphasized in the text, it is that the medical profession itself must take the initiative in developing a workable program, not this writer.

Lastly, I wish to thank Dr. James Dalen, the editor of *Annals of Internal Medicine*, and my friend Dr. Marvin Weisbrod, for their thoughtful review and suggested revisions to the manuscript for this book.

Tucson, Arizona

Chapter 1
ARGUMENT

There is a tide in the affairs of men,
Which, taken at the flood, leads on to fortune;
Omitted, all the voyage of their life
Is bound in shallows and in miseries.

– Shakespeare

SOME FORM OF national health insurance is inevitable within the next five to seven years. The inevitability stems from the resurgence of double-digit annual percentage increases to health care costs, combined with more than forty million citizens having no health insurance and an equal number under-insured.[1] It does not take the proverbial rocket scientist to realize that when the combined totals expand from more than eighty million to, say, a hundred-and-twenty million—roughly 42 percent of the entire population—Congress will respond to the predictable outcry and initiate a national plan.

Moreover, as the overwhelming majority of persons over sixty-five years of age are covered by Medicare, Medicaid, or other health insurance, the percentage would be closer to 60 percent of the under-65 population. Lastly, bear in mind that the federal government already funds 43 percent of all health costs, which immediately raises two points.[2] First, the government already has more than a foot in the door when it comes to national health insurance. Second, the cost of these federal programs will soon become too expensive for existing tax structures.

Now expansion of Medicare to all citizens is sometimes cited as a cure-all, but it won't work. Medicare is a subsidized plan in which workers and employers are taxed to pay for *some* of the health costs of primarily retired citizens. Furthermore, it covers less than half of the total health care costs of its beneficiaries, which leads them to purchase expensive supplementary policies or pay considerable sums out of pocket. In addition, Medicare does not cover prescription drugs, major co-payments are required, and the payment schedule is so low that many providers refuse to participate. And those that do are permitted to tack on what amounts to a 15 percent surcharge. Lastly, and most importantly, the plan lacks the ability to control runaway cost inflation. And where it does so by maintaining low reimbursement rates, providers simply increase fees for other patients.

The Canadian health care system is a more likely model, but it too has a severe problem in the cost containment arena. That system serves a more homogeneous population, which is merely one-tenth the population of the United States. Lastly, it is well known that Canadian physicians accept significantly less reimbursement for their services.

So here is the rub. A national health insurance plan may be inevitable. Yet in light of the necessity to control costs the plan could end up as one humongous health maintenance organization (HMO). And beneficiaries of *that* HMO would have no alternative, except self-pay to those few providers who would operate outside the system, as indeed happens in Great Britain. Worse, the federal government might leverage the plan to "improve" the profession of medicine through myriad schemes, just as it has done to colleges and universities with various sociological dictates on the basis of students receiving federal grants and loans.

In any event, the only possible way to preclude this situation from developing within the profession of medicine would be for the profession itself to take the initiative in shaping a national health insurance plan. Any plan, of course, could only be implemented under the aegis of the federal government, but it would be a grass-roots plan that solved *bona fide* problems of finance without beckoning a host of naive sociological ambitions. Thus the title of this book: *A Tide in the Affairs of Medicine.*

To be sure, the present administration favors initiatives by business and private interests. But there is no guarantee of their continuance in office past 2004, after which the medical profession might be faced with another Democratic administration. Remember the health care finance model that (now) Senator Hillary Clinton attempted to foist off on the country in 1993?

Furthermore, any such initiative would have been naive as recently as ten years ago. The medical profession had a reputation as reactionary, especially as represented by the American Medical Association. That is changing. The AMA and the medical profession in general increasingly acknowledge the need to overhaul health care financing, and certainly to bring an end to the many abuses of "managed care."

Actually, even if the professional outlook had been different, an efficient national plan would have been *technically* infeasible ten years ago. Computer science had not yet attained an adequate level of capability.

But in the last decade, the progress has been astronomical. For example, an Internet search engine can screen more than three *billion* web-sites *worldwide* to find all sites relevant to any stated criteria in less than one second. And do so while countless millions of users are logged in.

Also keep in mind that any national health insurance plan is insurance. It is not a health care system *per se*, except insofar as it makes health care services available to people currently without access. This limitation especially favors maximum use of automation, as it would be based primarily on mathematics and demographics, not the subjective aspects of medicine. If anything, our exceptional technical capability is the source of a different problem, namely the increasing loss of privacy, which will be addressed in a later chapter.

Still, the crucial question is: Will the medical profession take the initiative to develop a workable national health insurance plan? And if so, does it have the clout to ensure it remains workable? The second question is easier to answer than the first, and clearly in the affirmative. That is to say, if the federal government attempted to undermine the system for whatever reasons, the medical profession could simply withhold its services—except in life-threatening cases—until the threat subsided. There is no way to replace doctors as if they were air traffic controllers. However, this extreme measure is so distasteful that it is mentioned only once more in this book.

To continue, then, the balance of the text addresses the above argument in detail, in five sections of three chapters each. The first section—FACTORS—reviews the relevant facts, combined with the undercurrents and issues that must be addressed, if not resolved, in order to make any plan work.

The second section—EFFICACY—examines the nature of systems, then develops a generic model for a plan, complete with a host of potential options, supported by an appendix on some of the more technical aspects of an analytical computer model. It concludes with a consideration of governance issues, especially that of preventing the profession of medicine from ever again being subverted by the whims of claim processors.

The third section—COVERAGE—begins with a review of the most likely coverages, few of which generate controversy. Next, we turn to consider a few controversial procedures, both in terms of medicine itself and ethics. The third chapter in this section is reserved for the subject of mental health because there is no clear dividing line between orthodoxy and controversy. Indeed, the collective philosophy of mental health care is itself schizophrenic.

The fourth section—PINCERS—looks at privacy issues, fraud and malpractice, the last two being a source of major, and for the most part avoidable costs, both direct and indirect.

The fifth section—POLITY—reviews the propensities and problems of the federal government, followed by a chapter summarizing the likely positions of relevant factions of the polity regarding national health insurance. The concluding chapter then essays the implications of the challenge facing the medical profession, not only in its own environment but for other professions as well.

So much for structure. Let me reiterate the overarching theme of this book in graphical terms, namely that if the medical profession fails to take the initiative to maintain and preserve its professionalism, the federal government will eventually reduce it to *de facto* employee status. How? A single example should suffice, one that focuses on the most contentious issue in the whole of medicine, namely, abortion. And for the purpose of argument, it does not matter if the reader supports, opposes, or is indifferent to abortion.

On January 22nd, 2002, both the American Civil Liberties Union and Merger-Watch released reports—arguably preparatory to filing suit—advocation that Catholic hospitals be forced to provide voluntary abortions. The supposed grounds are that such hospitals receive federal funds (if only in the form of Medicare and Medicaid payments), hence they must "play by the public rules." Now, regardless of the reader's view of abortion, it is in fact that the Roman Catholic Church—and its 618 U.S. hospitals with 16 percent of all hospital beds—considers abortion to be murder. Hence if they are required to provide abortions, it would tantamount to ordering them to commit what *they* believe to be a form of murder.

If that were realized, all other dictates would easily sail through. The Republican party, of course, would fight this process tooth and nail, but in all likelihood the Democratic party will embrace it, as they did with so-called partial-birth abortions. Now anyone who sees a video of that procedure will inevitably realize that partial-birth abortions are tantamount to murder. And sooner or later, the Democrats will return to political power.

In conclusion, and as we note in Deuteronomy 31:19, Moses is recorded as saying to his fellow Israelites that he has set before them life and death, blessing and curse; advising them to choose life. Well, the profession of medicine has a life, so the question is whether that profession will take the initiative to maintain that life.

PART I
FACTORS

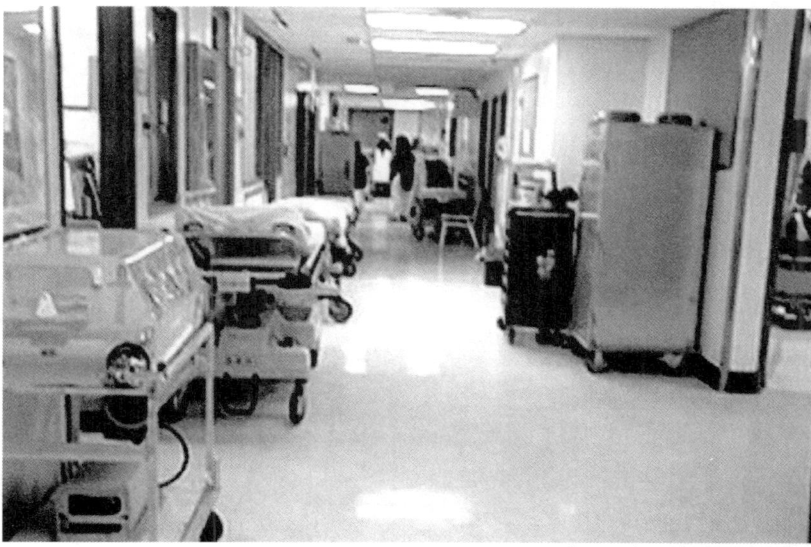

Courtesy: Long Island Jewish Hospital.

In many areas of the country, the hospital emergency room has become a clinic of last resort for the uninsured. And if lawsuits filed against the parent hospitals are any clue, these facilities often discharge such patients before they are stabilized. Perhaps more than any other single factor, this illustrates the need for national health insurance.

Chapter 2
FACTS

I only took the regular course . . .the different branches of Arithmetic—Ambition, Distraction, Uglification, and Derision.

– Lewis Carroll
Alice in Wonderland

THIS CHAPTER SUMMARIZES what are arguably the fourteen most significant, essentially verifiable facts or factors that must be considered in developing any national health care insurance plan. In every case, the reason or reasons for its significance are delineated.

OVERALL HEALTH CARE COSTS AND FUNDING

Distribution of costs. Not all health care costs—with or without co-payments—can be subsumed under a single plan, at least not with any degree of practicality. No insurance policy or program currently in effect, with the limited exception of the *collective* coverage for the extremely indigent under various Medicaid programs, attempts to be that comprehensive. Hence, it is critical to identify the total costs that would likely be included in any national plan, if for no other reason that such sum is the dollar figure that must be funded. Table 1 provides the summary data, with two linked caveats that can only be roughly estimated at this time. They are a one-time reduction in costs by elimination of most insurance overhead and profits and the offsetting increase of additional services that will be sought by consumers presently without adequate coverage.

Distribution of payers. The national health care bill is funded from many sources, some of which are funded from yet other sources, especially taxes, other than direct case payment or premium. The significance is three-fold. First, insofar as these sources are to be subsumed under a national plan, they must be redirected into a single "pot." Second, it should be obvious that the government—especially the federal government—is already the largest single payer. Third, many of these payers would no longer be necessary, particularly commercial insurance companies. Table 2 summarizes the relevant data.

Table 1. Distribution of health care costs

Category 1999	Cost	Percent
Hospitals	$390,900,000,000	32.3%
Physicians	69,400,000,000	22.3%
Dentistry	56,000,000,000	4.6%
Other professional services	71,000,000,000	5.9%
Home health care	31,000,000,000	2.6%
Drugs/other medical non-durables	130,300,000,000	10.8%
Vision products/medical durables	16,900,000,000	1.4%
Nursing home care	90,000,000,000	7.4%
Government overhead	72,000,000,000	5.9%
Government public health	41,000,000,000	3.4%
Medical research	22,200,000,000	1.8%
Facilities construction	17,600,000,000	1.5%
Total	$1,210,600,000,000	100.0%

Note: numbers may not total exactly due to rounding.

Source: Centers for Medicare and Medicaid, Web-site: <www.hcfa.gov>; Table 2. National Health Expenditures.

Table 2. Sources of funds for health care costs

Source	1999 Data	Percent
Government	$548,000,000,000	45.3%
Federal	$384,600,000,000	31.8%
State and local	$163,900,000,000	13.5%
Private	$587,700,000,000	48.6%
Insurance	$401,200,000,000	33.2%
Out-of-pocket	$186,500,000,000	16.4%
Other	$74,000,000,000	6.1%
Total	$1,210,000,000,00	100.0%

Source: Centers for Medicare and Medicaid, web-site: <www.hcfa.gov>; Table 3. National Health Expenditures.

Urban vs. suburban vs. rural resources. The importance of this factor arises from the fact that national health insurance is not the same thing as a national health care system, such as found in Great Britain where the government can more or less prescribe where providers are to be located. What is feasible in the United States is to offer financial incentives for providers to seek out or remain in less desirable areas. However, the worthy goal of improving the distribution of providers must be hedged by three limitations:

- Rural areas are decreasing in population, and size for that matter as metropolitan areas continue to expand into the countryside

- Rural areas tend to have small hospitals, which have the lowest occupancy rates, hence are more prone to be closed than are metropolitan-area hospitals.

- Hospital stays are much shorter than they used to be, and far more sophisticated in a technological sense. That is, any attempt to increase the number of rural hospitals, and to bring them up to par with major urban hospitals, is an unaffordable luxury.

PROVIDER/SUPPLIER DATA

Hospital occupancy and income. Hospitals absorb the largest single slice of the health care dollar, and there are only 5850 or so of them operating, compared to roughly 700,000 physicians.[1] Moreover, a substantial portion of physician income is derived from their work in hospitals. Across the country, the average occupancy rate is 66.1 percent, with said rates increasing in direct proportion to number of beds.[2]

Moreover, and contrary to popular opinion, these occupancy rates are decreasing, from about 76 percent in 1990 to the current rate, despite the closure of more than a thousand hospitals during the same period of time. Hence, the need to limit hospital beds remains as severe as it once was, if not more so. On the other hand, as the average intensity of care required per patient day increases, largely as a result of shorter hospital stays and an aging population, it's a safe assumption that nursing staffs will have to be increased, raising per diem costs even higher.

Distribution of medical specialties. To no one's surprise, graduates of medical schools tend to gravitate to the medical specialties, if for no other reasons than higher incomes and more prestige. In response, medical schools have done much to encourage graduates to pursue family practice and added board certification to that specialty, having long ago scuttled the name "general practice." But, as mentioned, the governance of any national health insurance plan will create financial incentives to reallocate the distribution of medical specialities. In turn, this will likely generate resistance from the higher paid physicians, especially those who are earning four and five times what the average family practitioner earns. In any event, table 3 depicts the current distribution of medical specialties.

Table 3. Distribution of medical specialties

General Medicine		**Surgeons (continued)**	
Internal medicine	17.0%	Ontolaryngology	1.2%
Family practice	10.7%	Other surgical specialties	1.8%
Pediatrics	7.5%		
Obstetrics and gynecology	5.2%	**Other Specialties**	
Cardiovascular specialties	2.7%	Anesthesiology	4.4%
Dermatology	1.2%	Radiology	4.2%
Gastroenterology	1.3%	Emergency medicine	2.7%
Pulmonary and allergy	1.4%	Neurology	1.6%
		Occupational & rehabilitation	1.2%
Surgeons		Pathology (including forensic)	2.5%
General surgery	5.4%	Psychiatry	5.9%
Orthopedic surgery	3.0%	Other specialties	1.0%
Ophthalmology	2.3%	Unspecified or Inactive	14.1%
Urological surgery	1.3%		

Source: American Medical Association, web-site: <www.ama-assn.ord/ama/pub>

Physician income. It is high and perhaps has reached the saturation point. Hence, one of the critical aspects of achieving workable national health insurance is adequate but not excessive reimbursement. Indeed, in order to give the appearance of modesty, the AMA recently included the earnings of salaried physicians to re-compute the overall average. The average income now reported is $190,000 (for male physicians in practice between 5 and 19 years), which must be significantly increased to get a truer picture of fee-for-service physicians.[3]

Insurance companies and their profits. The profits made by commercial insurance companies, as well as administrative costs to include Blue Cross and Blue Shield, are enormous, especially compared to the almost negligible administrative cost incurred by Medicare, which is roughly 2.5 percent.[4] Clearly, here is a prime target for reducing costs, not to mention eliminating the problem of refusing insurance coverage or only offering it at prohibitive cost to individuals with preexisting conditions or even merely the propensities for disease.

Pharmaceutical company profits. While many insurance plans do not cover pharmaceuticals, or only a small percentage thereof, it's a safe bet that any national plan will include this benefit. The problem is the enormous—some would say obscene—profits made by insurance companies (notwithstanding recent policy changes at Pfizer and other companies to subsidize costs for low-income families). Ten years ago, *Consumer Reports* went so far as to state that the profit motivation dominates over medical necessity and needs.[5] Perhaps the best way to illustrate this is by comparison with costs of the same drug in Canada versus the United States (in U.S. dollars), as done in table 4:

Table 4. Retail cost of pharmaceuticals: United States versus Canada

Pharmaceutical	Dose X Quantity	Price		% Increase
		U.S.	Canada	
Claritin®	10-mg x 30-tab	$81.05	$17.53	462%
Celebrex®	100-mg x 30-tab	$51.59	$14.73	350%
Premarin®	.9-mg x 100-tab	$86.39	$18.64	463%
Prilosec®	40-mg x 30-tab	$209.41	$97.13	216%
Zoloft®	50-mg x 30-tab	$77.08	$36.24	213%
Zocor®	20-mg x 60-tab	$252.20	$97.12	260%
Albuterol®	90-mcg [inhaled]	$29.40	$10.24	286%
Coumadin®	90-mg x 30-tab	$68.50	$26.54	258%
Synthroid®	125-mg x 30-tab	$54.04	$5.96	907%
Prozac®	20-mg x 20-tab	$86.64	$37.83	229%
Prevacid®	30-mg x 30-tab	$131.28	$44.00	298%
Lipitor®	20-mg x 60-tab	$206.14	$94.61	218%
Total		$1331.72	$500.62	266%

Source: Green Tree Press, Inc. in U.S. News & World Report, November 2, 2001, p. 33. The U.S. data was derived from three chain pharmacies in Erie, PA; Boston, MA; and Lincoln, NE. The Canadian data was from Consumer's Pharmacy Guide, October 1, 2001.

Fraud, malpractice and provider-directed excess use. As discussed in chapters 12 and 13, the combined cost of fraud and malpractice exceeds 100 billion dollars per annum, enough to pay for all the unmet health care needs of all the uninsured and under-insured. Under a national health insurance plan, fraud can be nearly eliminated, and malpractice significantly reduced by barring physicians from reimbursement when they exceed threshold criteria. Keep in mind that malpractice insurance carries exceptionally high premiums which physicians and other providers pass on to consumers. Furthermore, malpractice insurance rates essentially doubled in late 2001, making this aspect of health care all the more vulnerable to stronger oversight.

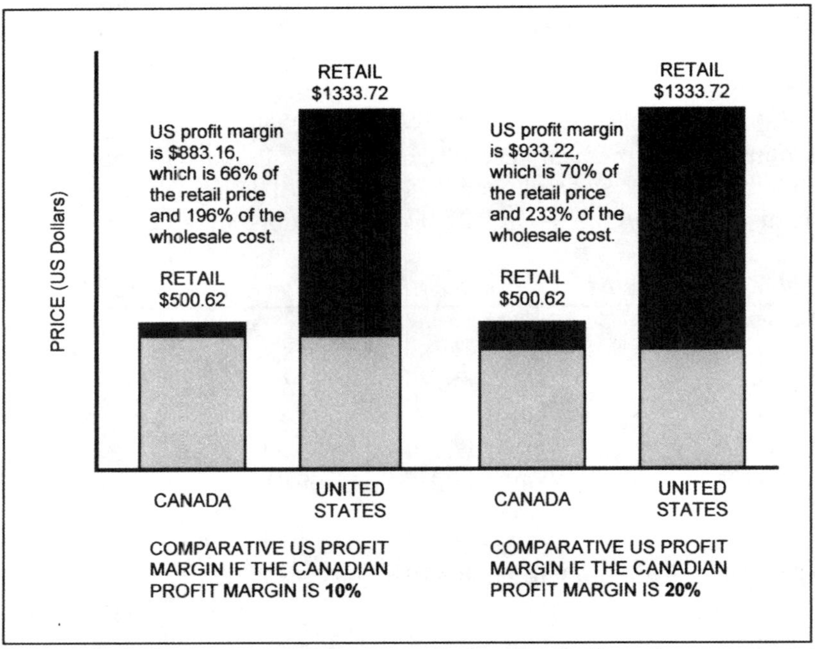

Figure 1. An indirect measure of pharmaceutical profits. *Profit on pharmaceuticals is much higher than suggested by comparison of prices in the United States versus Canada. The reason is that the excess cost is pure profit, and it must be assumed that there is already some profit built into the Canadian prices.*

MEDICAL AND PATIENT DATA

Distribution of medical dysfunctions. The complexity and variety of medical dysfunctions is beyond any kind of useful summary. Depending on who is counting, the number can exceed a thousand, although perhaps less than 10 percent of them account for 90 percent of all hospitalizations and doctor visits. What *is* necessary is to develop a universally-agreed-upon schedule—probably as a modification to the existing disease related groups (DRG)—so that processing in a national health insurance plan can be standardized, to include normal maximum and minimum days for hospitalization. Another requirement is to logically and statistically link these dysfunctions to facilitate detection of fraudulent claims. Any fraudulent-claims data filed by providers will likely form a statistical pattern that *collectively* lies outside the norm.

Last-year-of-life medical costs. This has a major bearing on issues and conflicts related to prolonging the process of dying versus life saving, especially when it comes to rationing health care in all but the most obvious cases. The pressure to introduce euthanasia in all of its many forms can be headed off by a detailed analysis of this data and the subsequent delineation of ethical standards.

Number of uninsured and under-insured persons. As mentioned in the opening chapter, the current number of medically uninsured persons hovers at the forty million mark, with roughly the same number under-insured, depending on how one defines under-insured. Just how much these numbers will increase as a result of accelerating health costs far exceeding the parallel cost-of-living indices is a matter of debate, but only as to degree. Moreover, there is virtually no debate that these cost increases will force increases in the number of uninsured and under-insured. National health insurance, of course, would eliminate the problem but not the related problem of escalating costs.

Patient-based contributory factors. This is extensive. And its recognition is essential to establishing the responsibilities on the part of patients and for significant cost-sharing, especially on medical conditions resulting in large part from addictions, obesity, and, for that matter, excessively sedentary life styles. This is not to say that any such plan could significantly reduce the incidence of these bad habits, only that justification for higher co-payments and/or for indirect funding can be maintained. A list of five among the more common factors follows:

- ***Alcoholism and drunk driving.*** The rough estimate is that some twenty million people are alcoholics, the majority of whom will remain so for life and who collectively cause half or more of all traffic fatalities. Then, too, although the vast majority of people consume at least some alcohol, it seems that at least half of all alcohol produced is consumed by alcoholics. If 200 million people in the United States drink alcoholic beverages, and 20 million are alcoholics, and we assume that an alcoholic consumes at least ten times more alcohol than a pure social drinker, then 20*10 is greater than 180*1. A significant new tax on all alcoholic beverages would therefore be justified.

- ***Illegal drugs and improper use of legal pharmaceuticals.*** There is no practical way to tax illegal drugs, but severe co-payments could be imposed on drug users.

- ***Nicotine.*** This is primarily consumed in the form of cigarettes, the reduction in the use of which seems to have bottomed out at roughly 30 percent of the adult population. They could be even more heavily taxed.

- ***Obesity, improper diet, and/or lack of exercise.*** This is the most difficult of all bad habits to deal with, if for no other reason that it applies to the majority of the population. For starters, any special taxes or graduated co-payments are ludicrously impractical. "Well, Mrs. Brown, your co-payment is $25 plus $5 for every pound over, lets see, your ideal maximum weight of, say, 140 pounds. Step over here on the scale, please."

- ***Reckless behavior.*** This ranges from negligence to the most wanton lack of judgment, and we are all guilty of it at least some of the time. And there is little room for imposing special taxes, except perhaps by special fines levied against reckless driving, including the operation of motorcycles without a helmet.

Patient demand for excess and/or unnecessary services. This factor arises from the disturbing statistic that more than half of all physician office visits are medically unnecessary.[6] The problem is exacerbated by public advertising of prescription pharmaceuticals with attendant demand by patients for various prescriptions. On the other hand, this statistic does not correlate with total health care costs for the simple reason that medically unnecessary office visits rarely if ever lead to expensive hospitalizations. Nor should we discourage office visits in the case of questionable symptoms. All that can be done is to collect data on what are deemed unnecessary visits and publish it.

Chapter 3
UNDERCURRENTS

I never saw an instance of one of two disputants convincing the other by argument. I have seen many, on their getting warm, becoming rude, and shooting one another.

–Thomas Jefferson

UNDERCURRENTS ARE CONFLICTING forces that cannot be resolved but which nevertheless exert a strong force on issues that *must* be reconciled for practical reasons. For example, a simple, easily agreed upon definition of justice has escaped us for millennia, yet our entire system of law and courts has been developed to manifest justice. However, the lack of definition does not create an impasse because the law is far more based on practical concepts rather than theoretical abstractions.

Health care, too, has its share of undercurrents, which for the most part are minimized when medicine concentrates on procedures and other therapies known to effect cures or at least palliate dysfunctions, without introducing more harm than already present. Still, the advent of any national health insurance plan will intensify these undercurrents if for no other reason that certain controversial procedures must either be covered or not. If these procedures are not covered, the only alternative is for individuals to pay at their own personal expense.

This chapter discusses four such undercurrents, all of which are highly charged emotionally, on occasion leading to murder. Various political machines and ecclesiastical institutions will all but fight to the death to advance their viewpoints. Indeed, one is reminded of the intense feuding and back-stabbing among the American patriarchs, so well described in Joseph Ellis' recent book *The Founding Brothers* and David McCullough's *John Adams.*

HEALTH CARE: RIGHT, ENTITLEMENT, OR SERVICE?

To begin, we have to ask is health care a right, an entitlement, or a service? This is perhaps the most fundamental economic question of our time. The reason is that the federal government assumes ever increasing control over various aspects of the national economy. The de facto resolution by way of various practical decisions will in turn dictate the degree to which the federal government exerts its clout over human lives in every social endeavor.

In specific terms here, the determination means the degree to which the government will attempt to manage and control doctors. And of course, to dictate what services will be included in the package of benefits, and whether the premiums are set per capita or whether they are based on a sliding scale or otherwise proportional to income.

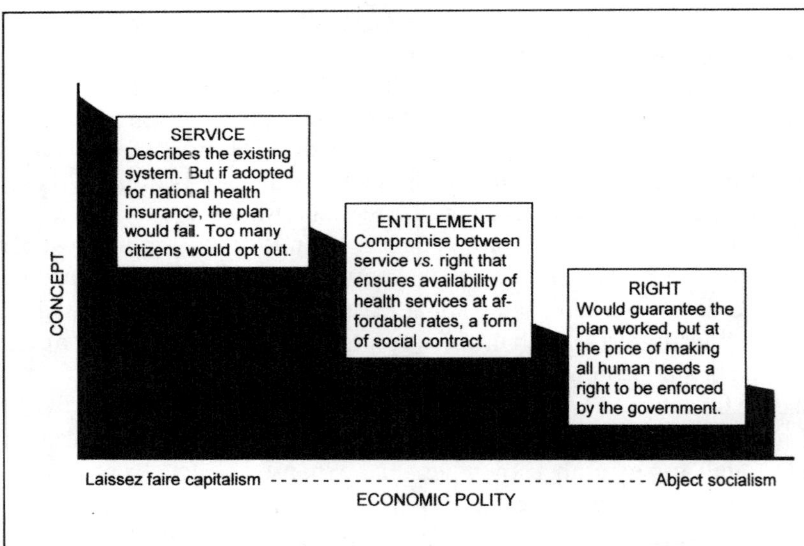

Figure 2. Health care: right vs. entitlement vs. service. Although the question of right vs. entitlement vs. service in any national health insurance plan may seem academic, the eventual answer will largely dictate how the economic future of the country unfolds.

As a right. If health care is considered a right, then the government must enforce its availability for all persons regardless of ability to pay, though as a practical matter it would have to assess premiums in some form, no less so than Social Security. The problem is that to date most formal rights are legal restrictions directed at the excesses of government, witness the so-called Bill of Rights (the first ten amendments to the U.S. Constitution). Moreover, most of these rights are restrictions against the government. Fortunately, the U.S. Supreme Court has consistently ruled that entitlements are *not* a right, beyond observing "due process" when denying a general entitlement to an individual.

As a service. Perhaps the best example of a service is the United States Postal Service, which citizens may choose to use or not, and if so, to what extent. At one time, there were few alternatives; hence the Post Office was originally a federal cabinet-level agency. Today, we have various delivery services, the telephone and faxes, the Internet and its E-mail, and messenger services. Now strictly speaking, the provision of health care is tantamount to a service, but we also see that left to *laissez faire*, more than forty million people have been left to fend for themselves.

As an entitlement. This leaves entitlements, of which the most prevalent example is the Social Security system. Each person who pays into the system (and to a major extent their dependents) is entitled to a pension, to disability income, and to surviving spouse-with-children benefits. Contributions to the system are mandatory based on income (up to a ceiling), and the benefits are calculated by rigid mathematical formulas. About the only leeway is the determination of whether or not a person is totally disabled. In this sense, a national health insurance plan would be an entitlement, in that premiums would be mandatory in return for guaranteed services. It would be subject to some co-payments, however, for the same reason that very few people can retire solely on Social Security benefits with any kind of decent life.

In sum, to declare health care a right would open the door to absolute socialism. For if health care is a right, so too is housing, food, clothing, transportation, and perhaps even vacations. At the other polemic, to presume health care is a mere service would introduce a fatal weakness, namely the collection of premiums or equivalent could not be enforced, thus degenerating the plan into economic Swiss cheese. This leaves only the designation of entitlement, provided that designation does not devolve into a so-called "right."

WHEN LIFE BEGINS . . . AND ENDS

When life begins is perhaps the most contentious issue affecting health insurance. In the absence of voluntary abortion, the issue would be purely academic, or more accurately, theological. But that is decidedly not the case. If life begins at conception, abortion is murder, pure and simple. If it does not begin until what we call birth, then abortion is merely a form of birth control. In either case, however, the embryo (or fetus) is not just another organ in the woman's body; it is a separate biological organism that, in effect, parasites on the mother for sustenance. Indeed, when push comes to shove, the fetus will starve the mother to increase its chances of survival. Still, that neither proves nor disproves the issue of when life begins.

Moreover, this issue cannot be resolved with any kind of scientific or objective rigor; it is too much a matter of belief. That the fetus gives evidence of life does not resolve the issue at all because those signs are purely biological, not fundamentally different than found in the lowest forms of animals. What makes the undercurrent even more contentious is anencephalia. Anencephalia is the technical name for a pregnancy in which the fetus has no cerebrum; not a trace. One pregnancy in two hundred is anencephalic, but almost all of them spontaneously abort, are stillborn, or die within an hour after birth. In the exceptionally rare case of a surviving birth (always on machines), not even the Roman Catholic Church contends that life—as it understands that term—is being preserved.[1]

The logical consequence is that if life does begin at conception, it must be entirely contained within the cerebrum. But the DNA of every cerebrum cell in any given organism is identical to that of every other cell in its body, and the various molecules and dynamics therein can all be reduced to permutations and combinations of inorganic processes. Hence the virtual impossibility of resolving the issue. And yet the practical ramifications must be addressed. Either a national health insurance plan must cover voluntary abortions or not, or only cover them under very restricted circumstances such as rape or incest.

This is not the same thing as determining whether abortions are legal or not. For the time being the Supreme Court has decided that they are, even in the case of so-called partial birth abortions. The decision required is whether (or not) any national health insurance plan should cover abortions. If the answer is yes, then politically speaking, the plan would be dead on arrival.

At the other end of the spectrum, we have the issue of when death occurs, brought to public attention by a handful of cases where a person has survived only in a comatose condition, reduced to a vegetative state, sometimes for longer than a decade. This can only be decided by legal means, and on a case-by-case basis. More significant is the provision of health care services to individuals with a terminal illness, especially when life expectancy can be measured in less than six months. So the issue becomes one of prolonging life versus prolonging death.

This is no small matter. As noted in the previous chapter, some 27 percent of the Medicare dollar is spent in the last year of life.[2] Keep in mind that the average *remaining* life span for those reaching 65 years of age is more than fifteen years. Worse, we see in Europe that several countries all but encourage legalized euthanasia, even in something less than extreme cases. What makes the issue all the more difficult is that it is not cleanly cut as in the case of abortions; no two situations may be identical, though there are obvious categories.

DEFINITIONS OF MENTAL HEALTH

The concept of *normality* in physiology is seldom controversial, and at the risk of oversimplification it may be thought of as the absence of any medical dysfunctions, or alternatively the maximum treatment and palliation that is possible for intractable conditions. In the absence of any *apparent* dysfunction or symptoms, about the only medical services necessary are vaccinations and their equivalents, and various tests to see if there are any embryonic dysfunctions brewing.

The same is not true for psychiatry and mental health. It is easy enough to define—if not diagnose—outright psychotic conditions, but what is considered "normal" in human behavior is arguably pathetic, even when it evinces a trace of rational thought. A more pressing issue is whether mental illness is primarily organic in origin or primarily psychological. If the former, then pharmaceutical therapies should be the treatment of choice. If not, then we are looking at psychotherapy as the primary answer. Moreover, we have the role of determinism versus personal responsibility. Are we the puppets of our genetics and environment? Or can we exert our will and change what would otherwise occur but for the exercise of judgment and choice?

These issues are sufficiently complex and will have an enormous bearing on what is covered and what is not covered in any national health insurance plan. The American Medical Association, for example, strongly advocates parity of mental health care with so-called physical medicine. But where do we draw the line between non-traditional, "alternative" therapies and out-and-out quackery? We'll return to this issue in chapter 10.

EFFICACY OF PREVENTIVE MEDICINE

Aside from vaccines, pre-natal care, and a few other procedures, the jury is still out on the effectiveness of so-called preventive medicine. The theory underlying HMOs was based on this premise, but the results have not verified it. If anything, the operation of HMO's seems more centered on squeeze-play money-making than preventive medicine. In the film *As Good As It Gets*, actress Helen Hunt utters an unmistakably pejorative comment on HMOs, whereupon just about every audience seeing it responded with howls of approving laughter.

Supposedly, we should be able to resolve this issue through objective research or at least objective analysis of the mass of available data. The problem is attempting to isolate and analyze the effects of various factors. We are all exposed to the same factors that are commonly associated with avoidable dysfunctions. A person who never smokes and has never been within a mile of a lighted cigarette may nevertheless develop lung cancer. So the ensuing undercurrent is not so much the extent to which bad habits and equivalent conduct is inimical to health. We know what they are, at least in actuarial terms. Rather, we need to assess the extent to which such conduct overrides the positive benefits of preventive care. It will take a lot longer to obtain that answer than to implement national health insurance. Still, we could all benefit from an increased emphasis on proven preventive medicine.

One last point, and it is overarching. Does the reader really think that national health insurance is just a matter of financial mechanics? Does he or she presume that concentrating more than a trillion dollars in a single nutshell—the effects of which touch every citizen from birth to death, will just waft along happily ever after? Think again. Even if we limit the mechanics of the plan to pure finance, its tentacles will seek to ensnare almost every facet of life and polity. For this reason, and because national health insurance is all but inevitable, how we implement, finance and control it is more than crucial.

Chapter 4
ISSUES

It is entirely easy to settle any question if only one principle is involved. But the hang of it is that most questions, all questions that are difficult, have a conflict of at least two principles.

– Felix Frankfurter

UNLIKE UNDERCURRENTS, ISSUES relevant to health care insurance must be resolved. Yet, if the resolutions evoke too much emotional reaction, the plan will not work well, if at all. There are many relevant issues, of course, and most of them are addressed in various chapters of this book. Here we will focus on four of the more significant issues, three of which affect all consumers; the fourth, more than forty million citizens over the age of 65, hence eventually all citizens who survived to that threshold age.

APPORTIONMENT OF RESPONSIBILITIES

This is an outgrowth of the rights-*vs.*-entitlements-*vs.*-service undercurrent, and must be established if for no other reason than resolving source-of-premiums and co-payment questions. Can one do anything he or she pleases inimical to good health, then expect the government to pay for the consequences? As we don't have this policy in criminal and civil law, it is difficult to rationalize why we should have it in medicine. Such a mind-set means that one may use illegal drugs, become addicted to alcohol and/or nicotine, drive recklessly, eat to the point of obesity and/or fail to observe even modest nutritional guidelines, engage in promiscuous, un-safe sex, and fail to exercise; then say to the government: "Take care of me; it is my right that you do so." Suggested guidelines are:

- ***Responsibilities of providers.*** It is the responsibility of providers to provide services in a professional and competent manner, for which they are qualified and for which they will be reimbursed by the plan. They are not responsible for individual health per se, except indirectly by way of providing services, nor for managing the insurance plan.

• ***Responsibilities of the government and plan administration.*** The obvious responsibility here is to operate the plan with maximum practical efficiency, and to use any financial incentive opportunities inherent in the mechanics to encourage better distribution of resources, to reduce overall costs consistent *with ethical parameters*, to prosecute fraud, and to at least inform the appropriate local authorities of obvious patterns of malpractice.

• ***Responsibilities of consumers.*** The consumer is responsible for his or her own health, except for dysfunctions caused by problems or failings beyond their control. Even at that, the consumer is responsible for participating in therapy and otherwise adhering to sound medical advice, which may extend to enormous physical exertion in the case of rehabilitation.

SUBSIDIZATION

Subsidization takes two distinct forms: partial or full payment of the premium, and partial or full payment of co-payments. Co-payments are essential to keep the system from being used to excess. Out-of-pocket costs are "felt" more sharply than premiums deducted from wages or other source of income up-front. Subsidization of premiums itself has two variations: a sliding scale based on income or a flat rate in which all potential participants either qualify for complete subsidization or none at all.

The present system is both lop-sided and vastly discontinuous. The poorest of the poor have all their medical bills paid for them. However, in the next tier up, at least for those younger than 65 years of age, we find that a large majority are uninsured, or under-insured at best, and will likely be driven into poverty in the advent of major medical expense. The cut-off income varies by state, but it is universally low. The obvious solution is to develop a subsidization scale, as depicted in figure 3.

MEDICARE SUBSIDY

This is a special problem, one which is perhaps the most critical decision in financial terms. The Medicare program is already heavily subsidized, but there is a significant premium required for Part B ($648 per person in 2002) and the co-payments are high.[1] So much so that most recipients find it necessary to either buy a supplementary policy or join a health maintenance organization or equivalent plan. Now as it is impractical—if not impossible—to expand the Medicare program to all, any national health insurance plan must provide at least equivalent benefits with no significant increases to out-of-pocket costs and/or supplementary policy premiums. Any thing less will generate a storm of protest from the 40-million-member American Association of Retired Persons, the likes of which haven't been seen in a long, long time.

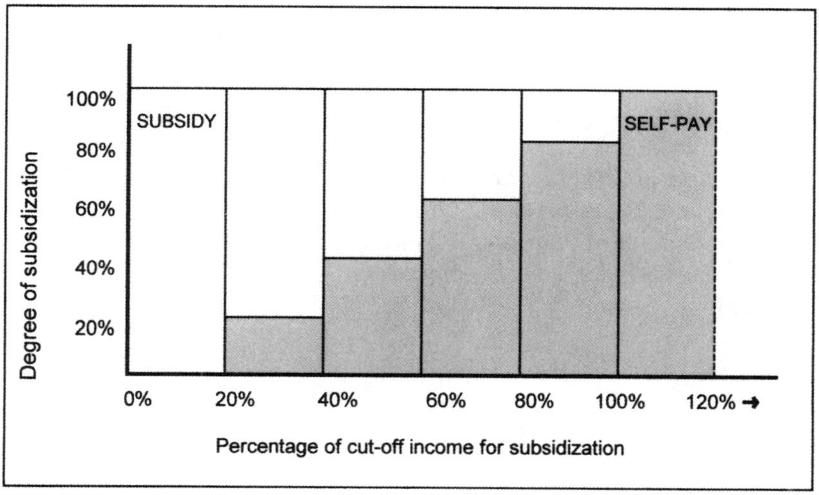

Figure 3. Subsidizing the indigent. *The poorest of the poor have all their medical bills paid either from the Medicaid program, or from Medicare with co-payments waived, or from various "free" clinics, or from the Veteran's Administration hospitals. But just above threshold income levels of eligibility, we find the majority of the un-insured. The obvious solution is a sliding scale.*

RATIONING

While the concept of rationing health care is commonly regarded as unethical, it has always been practiced, albeit seldom under that label. In point of fact, rationing takes no less than six forms:

- ***Costs.*** This is the most common form, in that where the cost is too high people will tend to avoid seeking help or visit an emergency room where they must be seen.

- ***General inclusions vs. exclusions.*** This form occurs because national health insurance cannot possible cover every medically-related procedure or service.

- ***Non-coverage of pre-existing conditions.*** This is a variation on costs and is quite common with individual insurance policies.

- ***Availability, distribution and/or and condition of resources.*** To no one's surprise, the density of resources is lower in rural areas and in inner-city slums, though public hospitals and clinics often compensate for the gap.

- ***Availability of hospital beds.*** This problem occurs only in a few local situations within the United States; if anything we still have an excess of beds. The same is not true in many other countries.

- ***Situational refusal to provide certain types of care.*** This ranges from the extreme of refusing to provide heart-lung transplants to end-stage terminal cancer patients, to restricting certain types of care to younger or healthier patients, for example, the refusal of the British medical system to provide kidney dialysis to older patients.

The crux, therefore, is not to avoid rationing, but to control the manner and extent in which rationing will be practiced, all the while attempting keep practical matters and ethical considerations operating in tandem.

PART II
EFFICACY

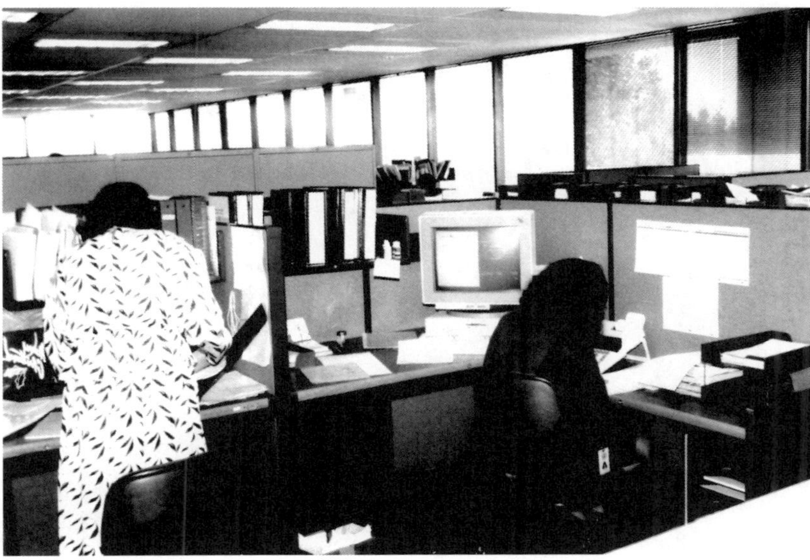

*E*FFICIENCY IS THE ratio of output or benefits to input or costs, whereas *efficacy* means the ability or power of a system to grow and sustain itself. For example, the efficacy of a fertilized egg cell verges on the miraculous. Yet, efficacy can also be negative, witness cancer, or for that matter, the ability of health care costs to increase exponentially. Although positive efficacy cannot be expected for health insurance, certainly the current mishmash of claims processing could use a little efficiency and at least some control over run-away costs. The three chapters in this section delineate how this can be achieved.

Chapter 5
SYSTEMS

Nature uses as little of anything as possible

– Johannes Kepler

A SYSTEM IS commonly defined as a set of elements or equivalents, organized or arranged to achieve an objective or purpose, or, once achieved, to sustain it. To be sure, this definition is so generic that it applies to virtually everything man and nature does, or ever did, or ever will do. Accordingly, no less a prestigious work as the *Syntopicon* of the *Great Books of the Western World* ignores the concept of system in its vast inventory of ideas, and the word seldom appears in any of its included works. The one exception being the title of the third part of Sir Isaac Newton's immortal *Principia*, namely "The System of the World."

THE NATURE AND FORMS OF SYSTEMS

There are two basic forms for systems, and two overarching modes. The first of the two forms is *linear* in the sense of *sequential*. In a sequential system, event A leads to B which causes C to operate in a certain way, which in turn may cause D to react as planned, and so forth and so on. Branching may occur at various points in the sequence, but that does not affect the definition. The branch a particular sequence follows is more-or-less predictable based on previous reactions. As such, a sequential system may be efficient or inefficient. Some fifty years ago, the famed cartoonist Rube Goldberg feasted on the design of ludicrously inefficient systems.

The second form is a composite of many semi-independent sequences that may follow any number of different paths among various nodes or elements. This form is commonly called a *network* but is more accurately described as simply *non-linear*. Perhaps the best known application is the Interstate highway system. This system contains less than 10 percent of the mileage of all major roads in the country yet it carries roughly 90 percent of all inter-city traffic.

The two modes are *pro-active* and r*eactive*. In the pro-active mode, the system itself is capable of growth, or that failing, at least the ability to change its mechanics to adapt to changing circumstances. The most obvious application occurs in genetics. Within this field a fertilized egg cell evolves into a complex organism that may have ten quadrillion cells at maturity, e.g., the blue whale. By contrast, the reactive mode can only react to stimuli or other manipulation, for example, message traffic management in a communications network.

MODE	FORM			
		LINEAR or SEQUENTIAL Operations proceed along specified paths, with or without branching. Branching is predicated on how the processing is to react.	Transition	NON-LINEAR or NETWORK Operation can begin at any point and traverse any set of paths among the nodes, either by programming or by human volition.
	REACTIVE Operations react only to external conditions, and only as programmed.	Simplest form and the easiest to develop and maintain. But human nature often rebels against this inflexible form. All health care insurance plans are linear-sequential.	Unwieldy branches	Very common, *e.g.*, all but dictatorial governments, and most transportation and communication operations. *Collectively*, health insurance plans are a network.
	Transition	Conscientious management		Inadequate pro-active design
	PRO-ACTIVE Operations modify themselves to accommodate change.	Almost a contradiction in terms, except when contingencies are foreseen and the system designed to meet them. Seldom found in health insurance plans.	Incompatible linkage	The most sophisticated form of system. It tends to occur only in nature and in a rare few governments. Too difficult for health insurance; too many contingencies.

Figure 4. Forms and modes of systems. *As complicated as systems may be, almost all of them can be subdivided into four groups based on two criteria: linear or sequential versus network, and pro-active versus reactive, albeit with transitional zones. The world offers literally millions of applications in each of the four quadrants. A national health insurance plan should be designed to move in the direction of the most favorable quadrant: linear and pro-active.*

The solar system, despite its nine separate planets and forty or so moons, is essentially linear in operation, witness our ability to accurately predict solar eclipses 20,000 years from now. By contrast, weather is non-linear, noting the difficulty we have predicting it twenty days ahead.

Not surprisingly, most non-linear systems tend are inefficient unless they are set in concrete, so to speak, which is literally the case for the interstate highway system. The reason is that for the same number of nodes, the number of possible sequences is much higher than for a sequential system, and that difference increases exponentially as the number of elements or nodes increases.

Think of elements arranged in a tiers like bowling pins. In a sequential system, the starting point is designated and paths must follow a sequential path, despite any branching. In a non-linear system, the path can start at any node and proceed to any other node regardless of where that node is located, like a CD player that can randomly play the selections in any order. For example:

Nodes	Tiers	Sequential paths	Non-linear paths	Difference factor
10	4 (3 legs)	24	72	300%
28	7 (6 legs)	5040	271,252,800	5,382,000%
55	10 (9 legs)	3,633,840	$2.307 * 10^{15}$	$1.306 * 10^{13}$%

Now let us apply this process to current health insurance claims processing to see just how expensive and unwieldy it can be. We take for our case study the federal health insurance plan for military retirees and their families over the age of 65. This is not to complain. On the contrary the benefits are exceptionally generous. The focus here is solely on the claims-processing nightmare, which typically arises whenever a new plan is tacked on to an existing plan that is fundamentally incompatible. This situation arose when military retirees were granted health care for life rather than being switched to Medicare upon reaching age 65. The claims labyrinth is as follows:

- ***Primary insurance.*** If the patient is covered by any insurance plan (except a supplement), the claim must first be filed with that insurer.

- ***Medicare.*** Any balance on the claim is then filed with Medicare.

- ***Medicare supplement.*** If the patient has a Medicare supplement, the remaining balance of the claim is then filed with the supplement carrier.

- ***TriCare.*** From that point, any further balance is filed with TriCare, albeit automatically in most cases.

• ***TriCare supplement.*** And if there is still a balance, then the patient may file same with any TriCare supplement he or she may have.

• ***Out-of-pocket.*** Any balance at this point is out-of-pocket, except as offset by cash-reimbursement-type policies.

Actually, the mechanics are more complex than depicted here because some procedures are covered by Medicare but not TriCare, and vice-versa. Moreover, the two systems use different fiscal years, which affects the deductible and whether TriCare will pay it for claims filed initially with Medicare.

Still, the above system is sequential, to include its branching. Indeed, all health insurance policies and programs are sequential in operation. The problem is that there are so many of them, and they are all so different, that collectively we have a non-linear system. Hence, any attempt to integrate the components can only end up with an even more complicated schema than Medicare-TriCare's competition with Rube Goldberg.

CRITERIA FOR EFFECTIVE AND EFFICIENT SYSTEMS

At least five criteria operate to make a system efficient and/or effective. There is a difference. Rube Goldberg's systems were effective after a fashion, but obviously inefficient. Conversely, a system may be highly efficient but ineffective. In London, a number of would-be riders complained that near-empty buses were passing them up—in queues of as many as thirty—at some bus stops. The official reply was "It is impossible for the drivers to keep their timetable if they have to stop for passengers."[1] In any event, consider the following:

• ***Meets needs without introducing major new problems.*** The story is told that a manufacturer of dog food went to great lengths to produce a superior product. Unfortunately, and despite intense advertising, it did not sell well. So they brought in the country's foremost management consulting firm in the hope they could determine the problem. After many weeks of research—at great expense, mind you—the firm came back with a tentative answer: "As best we can determine, dogs don't like the taste." What the needs are *versus* what management may think they are, sometimes two different things. And even when they are in synch, the system itself may inadvertently introduce new problems. In health care, the attempt to add catastrophic coverage to Medicare in 1991 led to so many problems that it was quickly rescinded.

• ***Employs mechanics as simple as possible.*** There is such a thing as oversimplification. At the extreme it earns the pejorative sobriquet of "panacea." But this mistakes glossing over needs and requirements for the simplicity of underlying mechanics that can adapt or be adapted to a wide range of circumstances without harm to itself. The common electric drill can be used for more than twenty functions (with the proper attachments), yet the basic design varies only in power and size.

• ***Takes advantage of interior lines.*** This is an abstract concept easily visualized by reference to a physical example, e.g., the Interstate highway system previously mentioned. *Interior lines* means having the fewest possible trunk lines or paths in a system so that resources can easily be shifted to meet needs as they change. Thus in communications networks, when traffic grows too heavy along the default paths, the excess traffic is redirected along less-used paths. And in this case, electronic communications move at nearly the speed of light, so the transmission delays in a conversation between two parties a mile apart, perhaps routed more than 50,000 miles up to and back from a geo-synchronous satellite, are imperceptible. In sum, good interior lines are nearly the same as having the fewest possible nodes—hence the fewest possible paths—in any system.

• ***Operates automatically, save for exceptions earmarked by the system itself.*** The more that humans become involved in routine matters, the more errors that occur, For example, most errors in Medicare claims processing arise from manual processing; the automated processing works very well.[2]

• ***Homeostasis.*** This means that within limits, the system is either self-correcting or that failing, sets the stage for corrective action. We all know that biological organisms are quite adept at this. When Walter Cannon first coined the term in 1932, it was immediately applied to political science and other human endeavors. A simple application of this in health care finance occurs when a calculated periodic payment is made based on past experience, which then is automatically increased or decreased when recent claims data warrants it.

PHYSICAL VERSUS HUMAN VERSUS ECONOMIC SYSTEMS

The distinctions among physical, human, and economic systems are crucial because they seldom operate well in tandem. Now health care and medicine obviously combine all three categories, and so we find ourselves in a bind.

Physical systems are the easiest to understand, notwithstanding the incredible complexity of the most sophisticated applications, *e.g.*, human physiology. Easiest, because no matter how complex a physical system may be, its inner workings and hidden mechanisms eventually yield their secrets to persistent analysis and experimentation. We know infinitely more about the human body than we did a hundred years ago, and it is a safe assumption that *eventually* we will understand all there is to know about it. Physically, at least.

Human systems, apart from the fact that human beings have physical bodies, have one overwhelming difference with physical systems, and that is the ability of each element—each person—to exert his or her volition, thus thwarting the intent of any imposed social system. Still, on a group basis, human behavior seems more predictable despite individual preferences, hence many social systems work well despite efficiencies.

The last category—economic systems—is a strange breed. In small applications economic systems operate closer to sequential physical systems. For example, the error rate in credit card billing is probably less than 1 entry per 10,000, and even fewer in bank statements. On a larger scale, however, we have something akin to weather. Alan Greenspan, as chairman of the Federal Reserve Board, is reputed to have said that the Board specializes in "precision guessing."

In the case of health care, we have a loose social system that aside from psychiatry and psychotherapy works on purely physical systems under the existing discombobulated insurance payment system. Thus it seems imperative that any national system concentrate on the economics, lest it find itself swallowed up by human emotions on the one hand, or become an attempt to regulate human physiology on the other.

HEALTH CARE SYSTEMS

Now let us apply this discussion to building a health care financing system. For the most part it is the applied restatement of the items, and which serves as a lead-in to the next chapter:

• ***Develop it from scratch.*** The present system is such a hopeless morass that it would be the height of stupidity to attempt to merge the present elements or to find some better way of interfacing them. If the example of Medicare and TriCare discussed above is any clue, it would be fatal.

• ***Include a three-tier hierarchy of corrective measures: (a) toleration of non-biased bilge-water, (b) homeostasis for significant but predictable problems, and (c) intense, high-level review of seminal problems and potential major changes.*** This means to tolerate a certain degree of random inefficiency at negligible cost for the sake of the larger gains in overall efficiency. It also means to design the system to quickly identify predictable anomalies or problems, that is, predictable in general but not exactly when and where, which is nothing more than an expansion of actuarial science. For example, traffic safety analysts can predict the number of highway deaths over a holiday weekend with amazing accuracy, but not when and where they will occur. Lastly, and largely as a result of maximum automation of routine matters, the board of trustees can concentrate on policy issues and the coordination with various governmental bodies.

• ***Keep the government infrastructure at arm's length, notwithstanding that the system must come under federal aegis.*** This theme has been emphasized already and will show up again in subsequent chapters. And it is true that governance of the system must accept a certain amount of political compromise within limits. But to go beyond this would be to make physicians *de facto* civil service employees.

Chapter 6
MECHANICS

Concentration is the secret of strength in politics, in war, in trade, in short in the management of all human affairs.

– Ralph W. Emerson

IN THIS CHAPTER, we outline a model system for a national health insurance plan. The core of this plan is marked by extreme simplicity, from which the myriad, complex applications can be satellite, managed, and adjudicated without damage to that core. Also, we must reiterate the indispensable element of automated computer support. The technology required is well within reach and has proven itself numerous times in other applications. Still, there may be some fears about placing too much reliance on it.

Two factors mitigate against this concern. First, *all* health insurance companies and programs already rely extensively on computer support systems, especially Medicare. Hence, the new system would merely integrate the logic thereof, except much simplified. Second, the integration and centralization of these computer support systems provides ample opportunity for extraordinary security of the data because the number of existing data storage sites requiring oversight would be reduced by at least 90 percent.

MODEL

The model is depicted in figure 5, which has ten key features aside from aspects of governance which are covered in the next chapter. The simplicity is obvious and automation support is indispensable. The remaining eight features are as follows:

- ***Two-tier structure.*** The system has only two tiers: a single governing office and roughly 200 regional administrative centers.

Most of the regional centers will likely coincide with metropolitan areas and their close environs. The balance will cover larger geographic areas but with much smaller populations. It is tempting to consolidate the regional centers, of course, but each center would need only a small staff and it would be in close proximity to the vast majority of providers it serves.

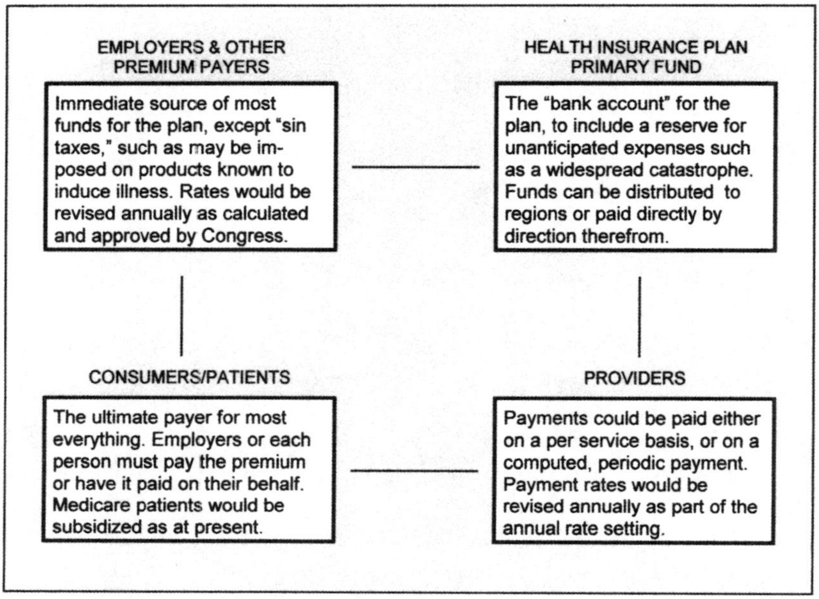

Figure 5. Generic model for a national health insurance plan. *This figure illustrates the primary flow of dollars in the proposed system. It gives the appearance of oversimplification, but that is because the system needs only two levels to operate.*

• ***Premiums.*** The major source of revenue will be premiums in some form assessed against every worker, in lieu of the Medicare tax, and virtually all other health insurance plans, to include the beneficiary payments made for Medicare part B. This premium must also be assessed individually against the self-employed and others. Whether the premium is scaled or not is irrelevant to this feature, though scaling would mandate intense coordination with the Internal Revenue Service to verify total income.

• ***Payment of plan benefits.*** The majority of the payments will be to physicians and hospitals, with roughly 10 percent *of covered* *benefits* going to other providers. They can be paid per claim or by periodic payments based on their recent claims history, adjusted each period to match exact claims history during the immediately preceding period, almost all of which can be accomplished in a fraction of second by automated analysis (per provider).

• ***Consumer co-payments.*** Every service would require a co-payment to some degree as established by the plan. For collection, the providers would be solely responsible. For the indigent, however, the plan would pay for all or a portion of the co-payment, and this may be billed to the plan if the patient is carrying an annually issued identification card verifying entitlement and what percentage of the co-payment is waived.

• ***Subsidization of the indigent.*** To the extent that an individual was indigent, his or her annual premium would be reduced or eliminated. Concurrently, the subsidization identification cards mentioned above would be issued. Computer cross-checking of these two features would be continuous.

• ***Annual rate setting.*** Of necessity, the operating cost of the plan would be assessed annually, with premiums adjusted accordingly as well as payment schedules for the subsequent year, preferably by calendar rather than federal fiscal year. And for practical reasons it would be unwise to make any adjustments more frequent than annually, except in the event of economic depression. Incidentally, annual rate setting should not be confused with changes to individual subsidization authorization, which may be processed at any time and as frequently as conditions warrant.

• ***Reserve fund.*** The plan would require a reserve fund to absorb any unexpected outlays until the effective date of annual rate setting. This is Business Economics 101, commonly understood by every person and agency except the federal government.

• ***Exception processing.*** As mentioned, the vast majority of premium collecting and payment of benefits to providers would operate automatically with computer algorithms to detect anomalies, patterns of likely fraud, and so forth. Also, special cases of extended treatment above norms and experimental procedures would be reviewed as exceptions.

OPTIONS

The above anatomy and physiology could easily accommodate decisions on a wide range of detailed issues. For example:

- ***Fixed versus sliding-scale premium per capita.*** This is a contentious issue, but in terms of operating efficiency of the plan it is irrelevant. The total of either method must equal the predicted benefits. A side issue concerns the premiums that would be charged to the unemployed, which except for the so-called hard core, tend to be temporary. Furthermore, married couples may still retain one earner in the family. Incidentally, this is one of the aspects of the plan that needs accommodate a minor degree of economic slack. The cost of exactitude here would far exceed any monies saved and would likely give the plan the reputation of being anal retentive.

- ***Fixed versus sliding-scale premiums based on age.*** The same argument holds here, though the idea of an age-based sliding scale seems to be overwrought. The vast majority of people live to past 65 years of age, at which point the Medicare experience suggests that premiums could not be further adjusted by age. This issue is similar to term versus ordinary life insurance, except that here the only termination of policy here would occur by death. Actuarially, then, it makes little difference if age-scaling is used or not, and using it only adds complications.

- ***National flat-rate, zoned flat-rate, or partially scaled payments.*** Scaled payments in some form are probably inevitable, at least for the foreseeable future. The cost of living in some areas can easily be double that of other areas, often much more.[1] Yet again, the decision would be irrelevant to the operation of the overall plan. Total premiums must equal total benefits.

- ***Flat-rate versus per-diem versus partially adjudicated payments to hospitals.*** The main choice is a flat-rate payment per diagnosis, or a per-diem rate with a range of minimum and maximum days within the range set for that particular dysfunction. The rate could be adjusted for payment of construction loans rather than depreciation, and a supplementary payment could be made for teaching hospitals. Objectively, the differences in these two methods are negligible, but subjectively one method may indirectly facilitate cost control than the other.

• ***Fixed percentage versus type-of-case co-payments.*** The underlying issue here is whether consumers should face higher out-of-pocket expenses for conditions consequent to bad habits. The problem is that such conditions can arise from good and bad habits.

• ***Control of number of hospital beds.*** This is a contentious issue that has been addressed for decades, albeit with mixed results. However, regulation of total beds under a national plan is probably inevitable. The issue then becomes if the plan itself would have that jurisdiction, and if not, it could always assume it de facto by refusing to reimburse any new "unauthorized" hospital or at least any additional "unauthorized" beds.

• ***Flat versus sliding-scale subsidization of the indigent.*** In all probability, some form of sliding scale will be necessary to overcome the current all-or-nothing policy, not to mention the fact that a single-threshold policy motivates people to drive themselves into poverty.

• ***Funding for health care for the homeless.*** If the payments are adequate, providers will much more likely be willing to establish clinics and services in areas where the homeless congregate.

ISSUES

Now let us briefly consider some of the issues fed by emotional undercurrents:

• ***Responsibilities.*** The crucial issue here is the extent to which consumers are held responsible for their own health, at least for those conditions which are known to result in major medical problems. That determination will affect the options chosen for premium and co-payment scales. And the more that bad habits are subsidized, the greater the extent the governing board will have to contend with escalating costs.

• ***Inclusion versus exclusion of controversial procedures.*** The more controversial the procedure—especially abortion—the more the governance of the plan will become mired down in an emotional cesspool, bearing in mind that procedures not covered in the plan must be paid for out-of-pocket (or privately subsidized by various foundations and charitable organizations for the indigent).

• ***Preventive medicine.*** The question is to what extent preventive medicine should be included as benefits, aside from vaccines and pre-natal care. Too much preventive care could overtax the system with only marginal gains to overall consumer health.

ONE-TIME SAVINGS

If the proposed system is fully implemented, then a substantial number of current cost factors will be significantly reduced if not eliminated. However, a good part of these savings will be offset by several new or increased expenses. We review the potential categories of savings, along with the new expenses.

• ***Elimination of most insurance overhead expense and profits.*** This alone will likely comb out at least a hundred-billion dollars. That is no exaggeration.

• ***Significant reduction in fraud and to a lesser extent in malpractice.*** Here is another hundred-billion-dollar windfall.

• ***Elimination and/or moth-balling of unnecessary hospitals and/or hospital beds.*** With an overall occupancy rate of 66 percent, which is significantly lower in small hospitals, there is much room for savings here.

• ***Potential reduction in the costs of pharmaceuticals.*** It is very likely that once a national plan is effected, enormous pressure will be brought to bear against pharmaceutical companies, but the resultant savings are too difficult to assess at this point. Also, the use of generic pharmaceuticals will likely increase.

Of the new costs:

• ***Increased subsidization of the near indigent.*** This can be estimated with reasonable accuracy, given the mass of existing income data.

• ***Increased nursing staffs in hospitals.*** This is the most critical problem faced by hospitals, witness the rapid burn-out rate among nurses. But if nursing staffs are increased significantly, the pressure to close any remaining inefficient or low-occupancy hospitals should increase proportionally.

• ***Wider inclusion of procedures and elimination of existing-conditions restrictions.*** This is so obvious that it does not bear further discussion except to point out the necessity of computer-based analysis of likely usage and attendant costs of the procedures will add to the benefits package.

EMERGENCY-CONDITION OVERFLOW

We also have the special problem of providing for sudden overflow of medical needs in time of emergency, and this could be used as an excuse to maintain inefficient or low-occupancy hospitals. But in point of fact, emergencies can occur anywhere in the country. It would be better, therefore, to plan on using temporary facilities such as the transportable hospitals operated by the armed forces, or to designate and prepare other facilities as temporary hospitals. Incidentally, the military's mobile hospitals evince remarkable sophistication compared to the tent city depicted in the film *M*A*S*H.*

Chapter 7

GOVERNANCE

Experience is wonderful. It enables you to recognize mistakes when you make them again.

– Anonymous

NO MATTER HOW efficient—or even efficacious—any social or economic system is, it still requires human management and guidance, if only for maintenance. Even the astonishingly efficient mechanics of the human body require occasional intervention. Else, medicine could fold up its tent and go fishing permanently. The critical point, though, is that such intervention—governance—should not be a substitute for inadequate mechanics but used instead to exercise judgment on matters which the system was never designed to handle routinely, except to earmark them. In this chapter, then, we briefly review the points relevant to governance.

Before we begin, however, we need to make one point clear on automation, lest it appear as a contradiction. Premiums collected can and should be deposited to a single account, though the actual funds may be invested on a temporary basis to gain maximum interest before disbursement. The regional offices can disperse these funds directly without first transferring them to local account holders.[1] By contrast, *most* patient data would be maintained only at the regional level, with only summary data passed on to the national database.

TO REVIEW THE BIDDING

At least four points are crucial to the effective governance of any national health insurance plan, aside from the need for maximum computer support:

- ***Arm's length.*** The governance of the plan must be at arm's length from the federal government lest it become subject to political manipulation for vote-getting purposes. Keep in mind that the plan will oversee or otherwise influence how more than a trillion dollars are spent, more than any existing government program, and it will affect the lives of every citizen and legal alien.

- ***Federal corporate agency.*** The plan should be incorporated as a federal "municipal" corporation because it would be analogous to a so-called natural monopoly.

- ***Clear separation of functions.*** The functions of governance and administration should be separated as much as possible.

- ***Toleration of bilge-water levels of mistakes and inefficiencies.*** By tolerating easily predicted and measurable levels of minor random inefficiencies, the management of the plan can concentrate of keeping the vast bulk of costs under control, not to mention the savings by avoiding the accounting for every penny. Even the IRS permits and encourages rounding off income-tax-return entries to the nearest dollar.

NATIONAL OFFICE

At the national level, the essential functions would reside in the work of the board of trustees and a small staff of experts immersed, so to speak, in the overall operation of the system. That is, the principal task of the trustees would be to set the parameters for the operation of the system and to maintain the index values for differential payments to providers in different cost areas of the country (and for incentives for resources and providers working in inner cities and rural regions). This is depicted in figure 6. In more detail:

- ***Premium and payment setting.*** This annual task would be the single most important function of the agency.

- ***Changes to exclusions and inclusions.*** If the plan benefits are carefully defined, and the decision is made to use separate plans for dentistry and long-term care, then changes to coverages will likely be incremental. Still, each change can have major consequences on its budget.

• ***Adjustment of factors in all categories.*** These might include differential payment schedules in different regions, payment-incentive factors for rural and inner-city providers, and subsidization factors.

• ***Overall security of the databases.*** While each region would have its own patient database, and the agency would have access only to summary data, it will be essential to maintain uniform standards of security throughout the system. Tight controls are also required to keep necessary transfer of data between regional centers. Please see Figure 6 on the next page for more details.

• ***Development of additional plans.*** While this book recommends separate plans for dentistry and long-term care under separate governance and management, a small branch of the executive staff of the national agency can work on the planning thereof, especially in light of experience with the basic coverage plan.

REGIONAL MANAGEMENT

At the regional level, the primary functions would be to disburse funds in payment of services, and to adjudicate exceptions processing. The most irksome problem would be conflicts with existing state regulatory authorities, which strongly suggests that most if not all regions be limited to a single state. This is especially true when it comes to the matter of regulating hospital capacity and relationships with state licensing authorities and medical associations. The most likely exceptions would be metropolitan areas that are still small enough to be served by a single regional office, but which spread out over two adjacent states. In more detail:

• ***Disbursement of payments to providers.*** The primary work of the regional office.

• ***Certification of eligible providers.*** Before any provider can receive payment, he, she, or it must meet established, published criteria.

• ***Checking on eligibility for degree of subsidization.*** This would be ongoing because the income status of individuals often changes, sometimes radically so. Incidentally, this is the one function that would likely require frequent and detailed coordination with other regions, and for that matter, with other government databases.

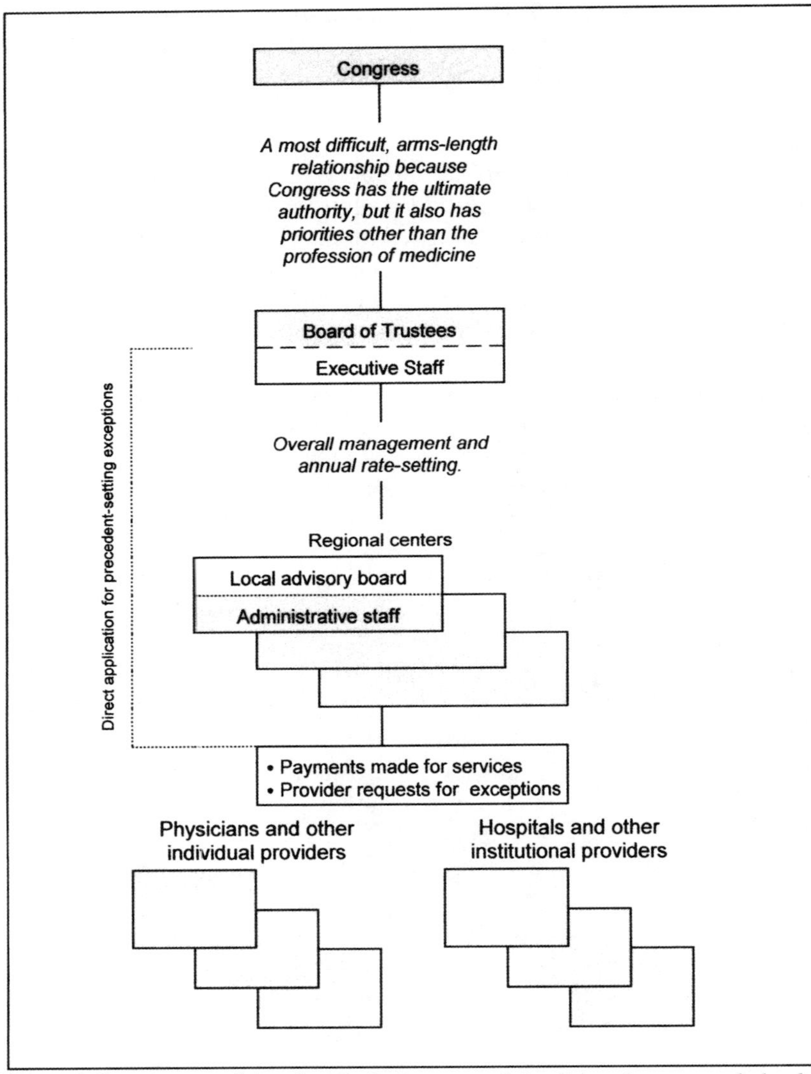

Figure 6. Governance of the plan. *In the interests of simplicity, the proposed plan has only two levels of management, and the functions and responsibilities of both are sharply defined and delimited. Moreover, the emphasis is on exercising human judgment when exceptions arise rather than micro-management of routine matters.*

• ***Detection of fraud and possible patterns of malpractice.*** Only the regional offices would have the data necessary for this task.

EXCEPTION PROCESSING

At the regional level, exception-processing should be limited to such matters as authorizing an extended hospital stay above the maximum limit and for waiving co-payment prerequisites in exceptional cases. For cases that would set precedents, exception processing should restricted to the national level, where a small office staffed by professionals can make decisions within minutes if necessary, and immediately notify the regional offices of the ruling and update codes.

MEMBERSHIP OF THE NATIONAL BOARD OF TRUSTEES

The membership of that board would be established by Congress, but initially the following might be considered as ex officio members:

• Secretary of the Department of Health & Human Services

• Executive Director of the American Medical Association

• Executive Director of the American Hospital Association

• Executive Director of the American Association of Retired Persons

• President of the American Federation of Labor-Congress of Industrial Organizations (AFL-CIO)

• Executive Director of Consumers Union, or similar consumer group.

• Executive Director of the U.S. Chamber of Commerce, or similar organization designated by Congress.

For the appointed members, we might consider:

• Two individuals, one each appointed by the U.S. Senate and the U.S. House of Representatives respectively (neither serving nor employed by Congress). During even-numbered years the appointee from the House would be the chairman. During odd-numbered years, the appointee of the Senate would serve in that capacity.

- Two individuals appointed by the President without the requirement for Senate confirmation.

- Additionally, a non-retired jurist qualified to practice before the Supreme Court, and perhaps nominated by that body, should be appointed to serve (without vote) as legal advisor to the trustees, provided said advisor had not been in active practice as advocate or jurist for at least two years preceding appointment and would not do so during tenure.

The rationale for the ex officio memberships is to ensure a balanced representation of providers, payers, regulators, and spokesmen for employees and other consumers. Insurance companies are intentionally excluded as they would be competing for the business at the state level. Moreover, any individual who was or had been associated with the insurance industry at any time during the preceding three years would be ineligible for appointment and would be removed from office if such a relationship were established during tenure.

The rationale for the appointees is to ensure balanced representation from the legislative and elected executive branches of government without the squabbles that have evolved in various confirmation hearings. And as for the legal advisor, the intent is to ensure the presence of a jurisprudential scholar, e.g., a noted professor at a college of law. This would be important if health care is regarded as a right, however unwise that might be.

Now it is true that the ex officio members could outvote the appointees, but there are checks and balances. First, the approval authority for coverage and general indexes for reimbursement would remain with Congress. Second, it would take high consensus to get that *ex officio* mix to vote as a bloc. Third, either all of the trustees must seek a near-consensus for its annual recommendations to Congress or else leave the fate of the system to political whims. This doesn't mean Congress must buy the annual recommendations, but it does mean that if it arbitrarily or capriciously overrules them, the consumers and recipients—read voters—would perceive it instantly. As for tenure of the appointees, a single four-year term of office, with the four appointments staggered one per year, would be the simplest way to go about it.

PART III
COVERAGE

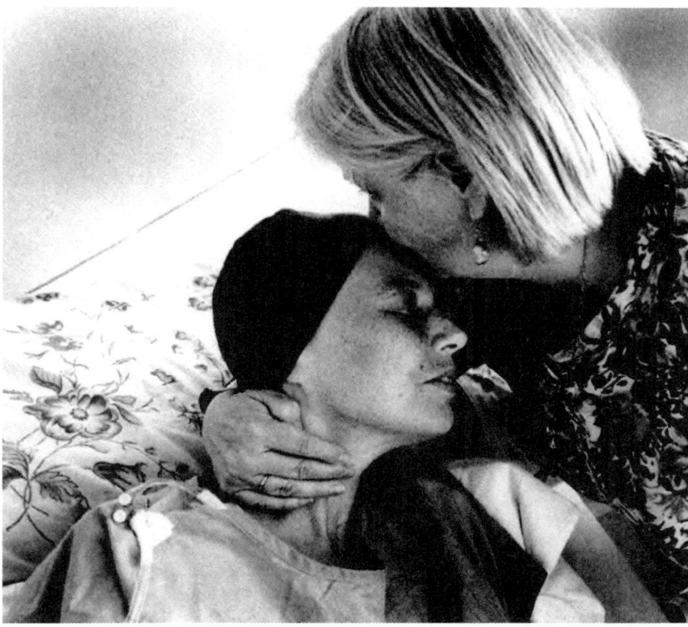

Courtesy: Roger Lymcyne

THE HOSPICE PROGRAM for patients with terminal illnesses is one partial response to the most severe cost problem in medicine, namely the concentration of expenses in the last year of life. But many physicians are reluctant to make full use of hospices, in part because of the understandable desire to prolong life at any cost. Yet even the Roman Catholic Church advocates "death with dignity," meaning to forego extraordinary medical procedures when there is no hope of preserving life. Still, such advocacy is no excuse for denying care when there is promise of improvement or at least stabilizing an otherwise degenerative medical dysfunction. This is at the heart of medical ethics, a matter that should underwrite any national health care plan.

Chapter 8

MAINSTREAM

Which of you, intending to build a tower, sitteth not down first and counteth the cost, whether he hath sufficient to finish it.

– Luke 14:28 KJV

IN THEORY, a national health insurance plan may include any number of benefits, the restriction being the need to pay for them. On the other hand, we easily find a certain consensus among the vast majority of existing plans, including Medicare, which more or less set the agenda for the majority of procedures that will be covered. Hence, the arguments tend to cluster at the periphery except for three big-ticket items, namely pharmaceuticals, dentistry, and long term care.

TRADITIONAL MEDICAL SERVICES

- ***Medical-surgical.*** There is no controversy here, except perhaps at the "extremes," and indeed the bulk of acute care costs come under this category.

- ***Obstetrics.*** The arguments for excluding this coverage are weak. It is included in Medicare for those individuals of child bearing age who are totally disabled.

- ***Rehabilitation.*** This probably should be included within limits, that is, short of when the benefit becomes custodial care.

- ***Detoxification.*** If included, it should have severe co-payments as the condition is always preventable by the consumer.

- ***Pharmaceuticals.*** Some coverage is probably inevitable, but a significant co-payment should be included. Moreover, inclusion will eventually motivate the powers that be to bring the obscene profits of pharmaceutical manufacturers to an end.

• ***Hospice.*** This must be included as it is already a major benefit of Medicare, and the vast majority of hospice patients are past the age of 65.

• ***Mental health.*** This is a difficult question beyond certain acute episodes. Chapter 10 addresses it in some detail.

ANCILLARIES

• ***Optometry.*** An argument can be made to include eye exams and related testing, but not for glasses or for surgical ophthalmological procedures intended to improve eyesight in lieu of eye-glasses, except when it is the only recourse.

• ***Podiatry.*** This must be included as an extension of medical-surgical. Doctors of Podiatric Medicine (DPM) are in fact trained as physicians with the obvious limitation of treatment and surgery of the foot.

• ***Chiropractic.*** This controversial ancillary is included under Medicare, but it is still anathema to the American Medical Association, even to some doctors who use chiropractors. The AMA claims there is no scientific basis for chiropractic, yet posits the full validity of osteopathic medicine.[1] Osteopaths differ from traditional medicine in that they also embrace if not practice chiropractic under the euphemism of "manipulation."

• ***Alternative medicine.*** This buzz word covers a wide range of practices, from traditional nutrition and other dietary regimens, to acupuncture, to homeopathy, to snake oil. To the extent any so-called alternative medical procedure can be established as efficacious in medical-surgical terms, e.g., acupuncture, it should be covered, otherwise not.

DENTISTRY

While it is tempting to include dentistry in a national health insurance plan, the arguments against it are substantial. This does not bar a separate national plan for dentistry, or more accurately, adoption of one of the existing if voluntary nationwide plans. Nor does it exclude emergency dental care as a necessary adjunct of a medical procedure, which happens in some accidents and diseases of the mouth and jaw. The reasons are:

- ***Different profession.*** Considerably less than 1 percent of MDs are also trained as dentists (or vice versa), and almost all of those few practice as dental surgeons.

- ***Cost and existing insurance plans.*** The total dental bill for the country is $56 billion, which is a mere 4.7 percent of the total health care costs.[2] Furthermore, numerous existing plans cover dental services, and there is less fraud and malpractice involved.

- ***Timing.*** Dental care occurs throughout life; it is not heavily concentrated in the senior years.

- ***Orientation.*** There is a much greater emphasis on preventive dentistry than in physical medicine, witness annual or semi-annual cleanings, X-rays, and examinations.

LONG-TERM CARE

Admittedly, the cost of long-term care is a growing concern, and it has driven more than one family into poverty and often into despair. Indeed, the total cost has reached the $90 billion mark, plus another $33.1 billion for home health care.[3] And we now see a proliferation of policies to cover such contingencies. It is therefore likely that serious consideration will be given to including it in any national health care plan, as in effect it already is under most Medicaid programs for the indigent. But that would be a mistake of the very first rank for no less than three intractable problems combined with the practical experience of the *Federal Long Term Care Insurance Plan* for military and civil service personnel (and their families). Still, these reasons do not ameliorate the concern, which leaves the alternative of a separate plan. And while it is not the purpose of this book to dwell on matters beyond a clear-cut medical-services program, this concern is of such magnitude that an exception is made.

The first major reason to keep such coverage separate and independent is that to a certain extent its use should be discouraged. There is a tendency of adult children to "dump" their aging parents into nursing homes when they no longer want to be bothered to care for them, notwithstanding the high cost. Once the cost barrier is removed, it doesn't take too much imagination to realize the consequences, especially as average life expectancy keeps rising. That might bankrupt the national plan or at least force premiums to rise to unacceptable levels.

The second reason is that the overwhelming majority of long-term care patients are past the age of seventy, and the majority of them will not return home again, or only under limited and temporary circumstances. Closely associated with this statistic is the fact that only a fraction of the population will ever be admitted to a long-term care facility, whereas just about every person alive will sooner or later be admitted to an acute care hospital and certainly visit a physician a hundred or more times during their lives. The significance of this is that if premiums were collected over an adult's lifetime, and allowed to increase in value by compounding interest, those premiums could be kept low. This would be in stark contrast to present long-term care insurance underwriters, who see it as a gold mine. A separate, non-profit national plan for long-term care need have no such orientation.

The third reason is two-fold: (a) the range and type of long-term facilities and programs is vast compared to acute care hospitals, and (b) many, perhaps most of them, and operate under less than ideal standards. Some would say that they are deplorable. The significance is that once the door is opened to long-term care, it could very well be opened to life-time custodial care for the severely retarded, the criminally insane, and what have you. And very quickly the trustees of the national plan would find themselves mired in attempts to improve the quality of the facilities and programs.

Not surprisingly, the existing federal long-term-health-care insurance plan operates completely independent of the Medicare and Medicaid programs, and the model proposed here is not all that different. Accordingly, and as depicted in figure 7, a separate, an effective, long-term-care plan would have the following features:

- ***Long-term contributions.*** As mentioned, if premiums are started early enough, and allowed to accumulate, the cost could be kept remarkably low. Keep in mind how modest contributions to IRAs grow into enormous sums in forty years.

- ***Voluntary versus mandatory.*** The plan should be voluntary, with premiums proportional to the age at which they begin up to the maximum age for enrollment. But for those who decline, it must be understood they will be forced into poverty if not destitution before any limited successor to Medicaid kicks in.

• ***Significant co-payments.*** Incentives are still needed to minimize "dumping." The insurance would prevent destitution or anything close, but there is no reason whatsoever for first dollar coverage. Moreover, such a feature would further reduce premiums, making voluntary participation in the plan even more attractive.

• ***Maximum use of home care alternating with respite care.*** Not all long-term care patients can alternate between a facility and home, but for those who can this feature would require home-care nursing to a far greater extent than is now available under even the best hospice programs. Still, as home care is considerably less expensive than resident care, it would further reduce premium costs without the odor of the plan "dumping" on the patients and care-givers.

• ***Quality control.*** The simplest way to ensure high quality is to set standards, enforced by a separate institution paralleling the Joint Association for the Accreditation of Healthcare Organizations, then ruthlessly suspend them from the program for at least three years whenever they fail of certification.

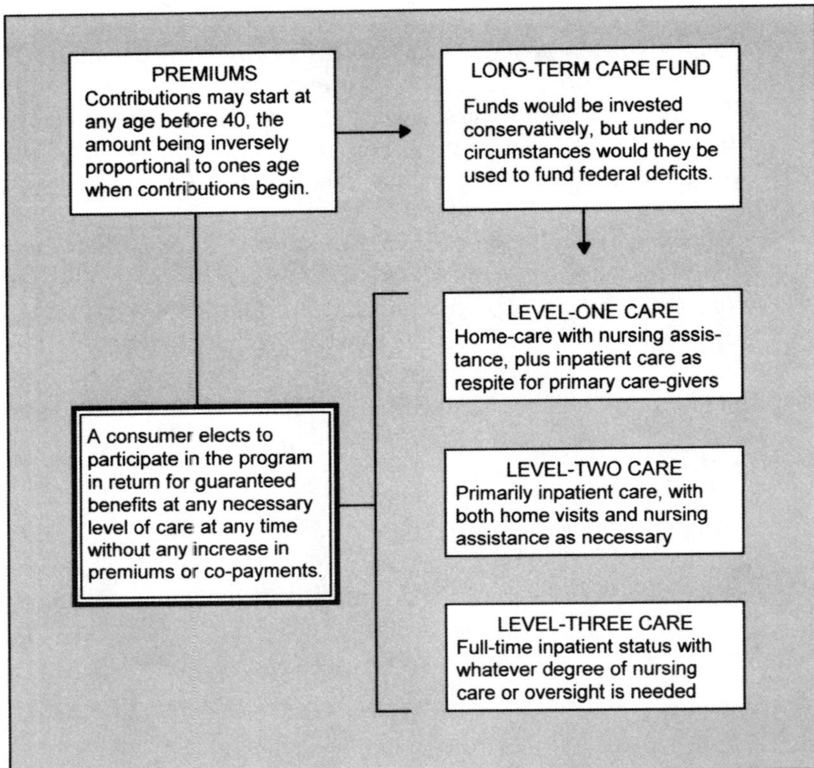

Figure 7. Schema for a long-term-care insurance plan. *The temptation to include long-term care in a singular national plan should be avoided; the conflicting parameters would lead to an impasse. This illustration depicts how a separate plan could meet needs while bypassing the potential impasse.*

Chapter 9
Periphery

For every complex problem, there is a neat, simple solution. And it is always wrong.

– H .L. Mencken

IN THIS CHAPTER, we review four classes of procedures that generate high emotional reactions, the first two of which could politically defeat any national health insurance plan if not carefully addressed.

BIRTH CONTROL AND ABORTION

Abortion is the most controversial medical procedure in the United States. During the nineteenth century, it was legal. Then it became illegal in every jurisdiction. Lastly, it was again legalized by the 1972 Supreme Court decision *Roe vs. Wade.* Yet while it is legal, few hospitals, clinics, or doctors will perform abortions, and more than one physician who specialized in abortions has been murdered by a pro-life domestic terrorist.

Furthermore, the Roman Catholic Church—with its 62 million American adherents as well as numerous Protestant denominations and Conservative and Orthodox Jews—adamantly oppose abortion except to save the life of the mother. Hence, it is safe to say that if and when a national health insurance plan is on the legislative agenda, and it includes payment for abortions on demand, that plan will encounter enough opposition to kill it, at least until the Democratic party regains power and shoves its agenda down the throats of every doctor. Is that the form of laryngology you want?

The same is not true for birth control. To be sure, the Roman Catholic Church is also opposed to this—excepting what was once called the "rhythm method"—but they are not nearly as adamant about it. Even the arch conservative Joseph Cardinal Ratzinger, prelate of the Congregation for the Doctrine of the Faith—and reportedly Pope John Paul II's right-hand man—has doubts about the doctrine, if only because of burgeoning world population *vis-à-vis* the limited resources of the earth.[1] Furthermore, the Church very nearly lifted its ban on birth control in 1968.

It would appear, then, that abortion on demand should not be included in the benefits package, although birth control counseling and prescriptions can be. This does not mean that abortion would subsequently be declared illegal, only that when obtained it must be privately funded. Then, too, various foundations, which would be relieved of an enormous call on their charity once a national plan is in effect, could offer funding for the indigent. Keep in mind here that the vast majority of abortions are low-cost outpatient procedures. And as a compromise, abortions in the case of rape and/or incest might be included in the benefits package.

END-OF-LIFE MEDICINE

End-of-life procedures will likely engender the greatest number of conflicts with ethics. And as implied in a previous chapter, the procedures range from those that merely extend the life of an end-stage patient for a few days or even just hours to those that can extend life for several months with quality. At the extremes, one permits death to eventuate with dignity while the other honors the sacredness of life. Certainly, this would leave no room for either involuntary or voluntary euthanasia, except in the limited and passive sense of withholding extraordinary medical care when it is virtually certain to have no significant prolonging of life. Accordingly, we can easily formulate two guidelines, neither of which is controversial.

- ***Informing and leveling with the patient.*** It verges on fraud for a physician to knowingly present a significantly more optimistic case on the efficacy of any medical regime for a patient who would certainly die without it, but who has very little chance of surviving with it, especially when the motive is to increase billings. The only practical solution is to require accurate counseling, which itself can be aided by Internet or other computer-based information written in lay terms.

- ***Honoring "living wills."*** This goes without saying, except when there are bona fide conflicts at law between a specific living will and legally binding obligations and responsibilities placed on the attending physician.

EXPERIMENTAL, NEW-APPLICATION, AND LAST-RESORT PROCEDURES

Last-resort procedures that are already standardized and part of the benefits package do not require exception processing with respect to any insurance plan. Other procedures in this category may be excluded from benefits, or excluded with respect to the condition of the patient at issue, e.g., the patient has a terminal illness, or the procedure will almost certainly result in death for that particular patient. In all of these cases, the fundamental issue is whether the exception will set a precedent, thus strengthening the case for eventually adding it to the benefits package. It therefore stands to reason that precedent-setting exceptions should be approved only at the national level, whereas routine exceptions are a matter best left to the regional offices.

The problem, of course, is the potential delay in obtaining approval, but that need not be the case. At the regional level, physicians can rotate on call to approve or disapprove the request, and he or she could be reached directly by phone. A similar case can be made for precedent-setting cases, whereby the call is made directly to a physician on call at the national level, with a copy of the conversation automatically recorded in the applicable regional office. The difference is that before approval could be made, a conference call would be required among relevant staffers, and for that matter a subcommittee of the board of trustees. The goal would be to obtain an answer at the regional level within five minutes, and, at the national level, within thirty minutes.

FAITH HEALING

Although the American Medical Association admits success with faith healers, it is only for psychosomatic conditions.[2] On the other hand, when parents of a child refuse medical treatment, and instead rely on faith healing and that child subsequently dies, they can be, and have been, successfully prosecuted for manslaughter. Hence, there is no justification for payment of such services.

That, however, will not stop Christian Scientists and others of their ilk from trying, if for no other reasons that some of their "services" are covered under Medicare. And it is true that scripture tells of many faith healings. Still, in this country we have separation of church and state. Furthermore, many of the "miracles" cited in scripture may be just so much exaggeration. Lastly, even if Jesus actually performed faith healings, he never charged for them.

Chapter 10

Psychiatry

> *I gave myself up to those feelings of eternity, which come naturally at the bedside of a cherished child drawing its last breath. At those supreme moments there is something in the depths of our souls that tells us the world is more than a mere combination of phenomena appropriate for a mechanical equilibrium wrought from the chaos of nature solely by way of the gradual actions of the forces of nature.*
>
> – Louis Pasteur, MD

THERE'S NOT MUCH poetry in an operating room; there can be to life. That, sometimes, is the conflict between so-called physical medicine and psychiatry. Unfortunately, under any national health insurance plan, that conflict would have to be resolved. Of necessity, any plan must have uniform coverage. Uniform coverage means reaching a consensus on what to include. That task is difficult enough with physical medicine. With respect to psychiatry, it's a major undertaking.

The reason is threefold. First, there are significant differences between physical medicine and psychiatry. Second, psychiatry offers a much broader range and depth of acceptable therapies and treatments for many, if not most, conditions, especially when the closely related fields in psychology are included. Third, taken to a logical extreme, the pursuit of mental health could evolve into socialism, where the government not only ensures that mental health care is considered a right but exercises the power to coerce individuals to conform to what is considered "normal" behavior.

That may seem like an exaggeration, but the incredible prosecution of an unmarried mother in Syracuse, New York, for the most asinine reasons indicates that the exaggeration is one of degree not substance. The case involved a nursing mother who mentioned to her case worker that she was having a mild sensual reaction while breast feeding her baby, for which common-enough reaction she was arrested as a child molester.[1] To continue, then, this chapter examines the major differences between physical medicine and psychiatry-psychology and then reviews the significance.

DIFFERENCES

For the most part, the practice of medicine is short term and where possible, aims at restoring the status quo. A healthy person need not consult with doctors except for preventive medicine and early detection of problems that may be without symptoms at the moment. By contrast, the practice of psychiatry and psychology are often immersed in long-term treatment, and agreement on what constitutes "mental health" is anything but a settled issue. Some schools of thought hold that what is supposedly normal behavior is inadequate at best; more pathetic than rewarding.

Related to this is the question of causes. Most physical conditions have physical roots, notwithstanding psychosomatic contributions and aggravations. Cancer, coronaries, and diabetes are not products of the mind. Nor are most accidents, especially when the victim is an innocent bystander. Sometimes, one's mental health may prevent physical problems from recurring, or more likely the process of recovery may go further and faster, but treatment of acute coronary conditions and diabetes is not the domain of psychiatry.

The reason is easy to discern. Most individuals are born healthy, and most of those that are not have specific, identifiable deficiencies. With reasonably good diet and living conditions, most of the healthy ones will continue in that state of health until they reach 45 years of age or older. Hospitalization is infrequent between the ages of 15 and 44, and much of that is accident or war related.[2] For immediate proof, examine any age-indexed individual health insurance premium schedule.

Mental health does not follow suit. It is the product of genetic endowment and a lifetime of experience and learning. The proportionality is the subject of intense debate and undoubtedly it varies among individuals, but few practitioners hold that babies are born with perfect mental health and that only negative experiences detract from it. On the contrary, the attainment of deep-seated satisfaction and equanimity in the conduct of life is difficult under the best of conditions. When an individual has struggled through a traumatic childhood, it is an uphill struggle, one that is often lost.

On another level, it may be said that physical health is driven by chemical balances and imbalances, by functional or partially dysfunctional nervous systems, and so forth. By contrast, mental health is driven by emotions, by perceptions and the subconscious, by the ability to clearly see or not see the relationships between inner drives and motivations versus outward events and experience, and by the affects, which range from the experience of love, equanimity, and cheerfulness; to hate, anxiety, and indifference. Thus many therapies in psychiatry and psychology are based on a conscious retracing of roots, from childhood if necessary. By contrast, physical medicine prefers to root out a problem as it exists, or at least controlling it. How it formed or when it formed is usually less important than identifying immediate causes. Even when it is essential to identify those physiological liabilities, the intent is usually to control relapses or recurrences.

Still another difference is the concept of "normality." That term rarely inspires much debate in physical medicine. It's a different story in mental health. True, it could be and sometimes is defined as the absence of psychotic or severe neurotic conditions, which thus accepts most neuroses and a host of other shortcomings as "normal." Still, the vast majority of mental health problems, as gauged by the number of patients and clients rather than costs, are not psychotic in nature. Moreover, the road to health often depends on the make-up of the individual. Is it grief over the loss of a loved one carried too far or too long? Is it chronic depression stemming from an inability to manifest one's *bona fide* interests and talents? Or is it excessive guilt over past mistakes? Or a lack of sufficient guilt or remorse over intentional acts harmful to others? In short, normality in mental health is an elusive term and hinges on many subjective factors.

To this must be added the much wider range of acceptable therapies and treatments in mental health compared to physical medicine. With many physical disorders, acceptable treatments adhere to a narrow path. True, in some cancers, surgery versus radiation versus chemotherapy are options. And the debate on how much surrounding tissue should be removed, especially in breast cancer, drones on endlessly. But when it comes to mental health, one only need read the various theories of Sigmund Freud, Carl Jung, Alfred Adler, Karl Menninger, Erich Fromm, Rollo May, Viktor Frankl, Jean Piaget, Erik Erikson, Kurt Lewin, and Harry Stack Sullivan among others, to grasp the range here and the apparent irreconcilability of the various schools of thought.

The obvious compromise is that different individuals, at different times in their lives, can benefit from different approaches. Still, some of the options involve low cost counseling and no-cost support. Others, like psychoanalysis, can take five or more years and cost $100,000 or more.

Further, the conflict over appropriate therapies for those conditions that are obviously disabling is almost as livid. Some professionals stress drug therapy; others, the one-on-one therapeutic environment; still others, family involvement, group therapy and support groups. Franz Alexander and Sheldon Selesnick, in their landmark *History of Psychiatry*, put the case this way:

> And the struggle still goes on to the present day. The role of the devil has now been taken over by brain chemistry. No longer a devil but a *deus ex machina*, a disturbed brain chemistry rather than a person's own life experiences, is responsible for mental illness. Whatever the cause of faulty brain chemistry may be, the new conviction is that the disturbed mind can now be cured by drugs and that the patient himself as a person no longer needs to try to understand the source of his troubles and master them by mental processes.[3]

Another key difference is that mental health increasingly depends on involvement of the family or loved ones as part of the therapy, whereas in physical medicine this is often seen as merely supportive. The reason is that those relationships may have exacerbated if not caused the condition. As a minimum, the support by friends and loved ones may be necessary to help the individual over the hump, so to speak, in the absence of will power (a concept that itself is hotly debated) to go it alone. By contrast, the onset of insulin-dependent diabetes mellitus is rarely a product of family life, though the patient obviously needs the support of his or her family and can certainly do without any ridicule.

Still another obvious difference is that while medicine is dominated by physicians the same is not true in the field of mental health. There are more psychologists than psychiatrists, and PhD psychologists are now admitted to psychoanalytic training programs. Further, physical medicine depends on physical intervention, be it the quick way by surgery, radiation or some equivalent; or by drugs, diet or similar. Bedside manner is nice to have, but most short-term patients will trade it for absolute competence on the part of the physician, especially in cases of surgery.

In psychology, however, something akin to bedside manner is critical. It goes by many names, among them "the laying on of the psychical hands." An even greater number of theories try to explain the effect and how it should be utilized. Some posit that the respect and love—in the most mature sense of that word—an analyst demonstrates toward a patient can instill a genuine sense of self-respect as the basis for any further improvement, especially if that patient had been deprived of it in their childhood, and hence this is the real source, or at least the primary source, of healing.

Then, too, consider the literature written on the subject. Books on physical medicine are seldom popular. About 30 years ago, Gustav Eckstein's *The Body Has a Head* was the main selection of the Book of the Month Club, and the Lewis Thomas anthologies of his own essays remain popular. But aside from various one-volume encyclopedias, e.g., AMA, Mayo Clinic, and Columbia University, there's not much on the layman's shelf. Not so in the field of psychiatry and psychology. Walk into any chain bookstore, and you will find at least a hundred titles. Even Freud's works still sell in the tens of thousands of copies annually. Moreover, while the ancient treatises on physical medicine are often a source of hindsight humor, the works of the Greek tragedians and Shakespeare seem to be as valid today as ever.

SIGNIFICANCE

This leads directly to the debate on the role of character versus disease, especially when it comes to addictions. The concept of character is based on personal responsibility for one's actions. The concept of disease, by contrast, implies factors which are beyond the individual to control. For polemics, the former says: "These are the facts and the law. If you don't mend your ways, these are the consequences." The latter says: "You are not capable of dealing with your problem. We are obliged to intervene to the extent that you cannot, or at least until that point is reached when can cope largely on your own."

Now obviously, when an individual is psychotic and beyond rational judgment, somebody has to intervene, although just what specific therapies can be forced on a patient is open to debate. Remember insulin shock therapy and prefrontal lobotomies? At the other extreme, no credible professional will advocate massive intervention when a family has a passively neurotic squabble over whether to go the beach or the mountains for a vacation. It's the stuff between where the potential trouble lies.

This conflict is sometimes brought to the forefront in the courtroom when a defendant pleads not guilty by reason of insanity. John Hinckley, who attempted to kill President Reagan, was adjudged insane at the time of the crime, and is still confined at St. Elizabeth's Hospital in Washington, D.C. By contrast, the same defense failed in the Jeffrey Dahmer case, and he was sentenced to 15 consecutive life terms.

Although incarceration in a penitentiary and a ward for the criminally insane may not seem much different in practice, that is tangential to the thesis here. If the insanity defense fails—and it almost always does—and the crime is capital, the individual can be executed. But when this defense prevails, the individual is no longer a criminal. He is a patient who can be released whenever psychiatrists certify—often with the concurrence of the courts—that the condition has been "cured" or at least abated sufficiently to let him or her return to a life of freedom. Fortunately, the number of insanity-defense cases are small. Unfortunately, to the extent that the insanity defense exists at all is the extent to which the state, and hence caregivers under a national health care system, could assume responsibility and forcibly place an individual under their control.

In all of this welter, then, we must ask: What are the parameters for deciding which mental-health procedures and therapies to include in any national plan? Economically, the categories are: (a) psychiatrists, (b) long-term use of psycho-active pharmaceuticals, (c) qualified psychologists and equivalents, and (d) short-term hospitalization for acute episodes. That is where most of the money is spent and to which most of the dramatic cases gravitate. But we also need to consider the ethical center of gravity related to personal responsibility. Nudging ethics and therapy closer together is no small task. Hence, it is in this arena that the definition of health and health care runs the greatest danger of slipping into absolute socialism.

PART IV
PINCERS

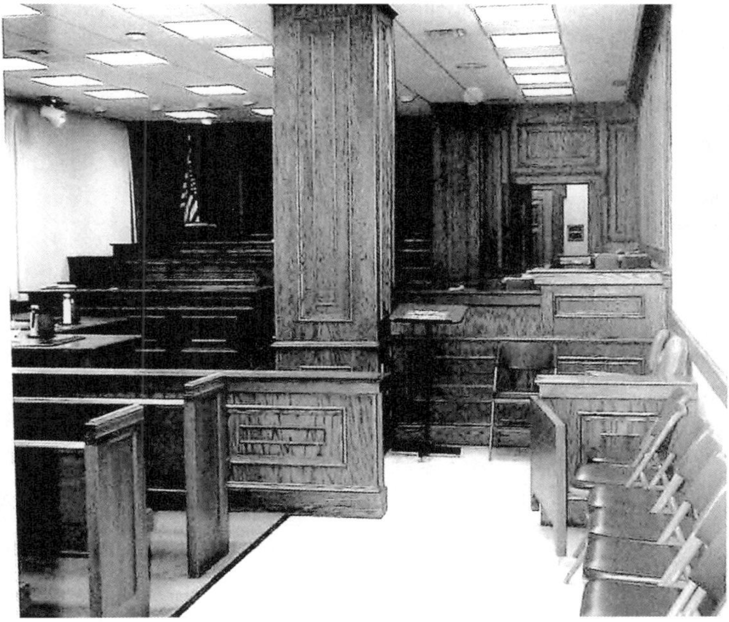

Courtesy: Mercer County, Pennsylvania.

WE LIKE TO comfort ourselves that serious wrongdoing in the practice of medicine is uncommon, almost an anomaly. Unfortunately, and while actual courtroom cases remain something of an exception, fraud and malpractice cost us in excess of a hundred billion dollars a year. These are major if indirect costs that would surely come under sharp focus in any national health insurance plan, if only by facilitating scrutiny via integrated, almost singular databases. And those databases themselves raise another specter, namely that of an increased loss of privacy. In this part of the book, then, we examine these three "pincers" at some length, starting with privacy concerns.

Chapter 11
Privacy

Disproportion is the root of all moral mistakes. . . .within most virtues there lurks, waiting to slip its leash, a vice in the form of excess.

– George Will

THE AGE OF automation has spawned numerous benefits, not the least of which have been spectacular advances in medical research and diagnosis and, in turn, more than a few computer-assisted therapies. On the other hand, this same technology has spawned major problems in privacy, for example, the misuse of medical data in job hiring and retention. Without a doubt, any national health care insurance plan would exacerbate problems of this kind and introduce several new ones. This chapter explains why and offers a few suggestions on what can be done to ameliorate these problems

NATURE OF THE BEAST

The root of automation-based privacy issues is the massing of data on an unprecedented scale, combined with ease of access to an ever widening circle of users. What makes this situation especially difficult is that much of the data is public information. Now there is nothing illegal or immoral about reading public information, or using it for legitimate purposes. Still, as recently as a single generation ago, the mass of this data was largely ignored because it was too cumbersome to collate or use to any marked extent. But now that it has become widely available, we sense an "invasion" of our privacy. Worse, it is easier to combine this public information with private data, with a concurrent slide into questionable if not outright illegal use.

This situation is not all bad. Perhaps the most dramatic example was the ease with which the federal government and various law enforcement agencies were able to identify all of the terrorist hijackers in the attacks of September 11, 2001 in less than twenty-four hours, and only a short time later to pin down the responsibility to Osama Bin Laden. Indeed, the ability of passengers on United Flight #93 to place calls made them realize that they were victims of a mass suicide, which motivated a few of them to attack the high-jackers. This saved perhaps thousands of lives, presumably in Washington, D.C., had the hijackers succeeded in their plan.

On the negative side, we have—among other items—numerous cases of job discrimination traceable to medical conditions. Even more prevalent is the denial of health insurance, or alternatively, unacceptably high premiums and exclusions for perhaps the majority of individual applicants.[1] Nor are physicians immune to this misuse. Consider the *CourtScan* program in Philadelphia, which tracks virtually all malpractice suits filed against physicians and other health care providers by patients.[2] This data is used by physicians to refuse to accept potential patients if there is any increased risk of being sued for malpractice whether merited or not.

LEVELS AND APPLICATIONS

While privacy can be "invaded" in many ways, most ways can be categorized under the three degrees or levels of severity. The significance is the corresponding level of protection that should be exercised to ameliorate if not preclude abuse, which translates into more specific measures when applied to health insurance:

- ***Low-level.*** This level ranges from use of data for statistical purposes without identifying individuals, to obtaining information on an individual that is either public information or which can be readily discerned by almost any observer. As such, this level precludes direct counteractions, which should instead focus on preventing decisions that would be inimical to patients, for example, rationing of services beyond acceptable levels.

- ***Mid-level.*** This level typically uses private data to discriminate or otherwise inflict an unfair disadvantage against an individual, be it in the form of job discrimination or insurance applications. In *practical* terms, the abuse may or may not be actionable in court. Still, remedies must focus both on restricting access to the data and inflicting severe penalties on those persons who violate those restrictions. And keep in mind that some discrimination is perfectly legitimate. Potential employees with a history of epileptic seizures should not be hired to operate public transportation.

• ***High-level.*** This level is invariably felonious, for example, blackmail in the case of venereal disease. Hence, it is actionable in criminal court and often in civil court. In some cases, fear of exposure and/or discrimination may cause a patient to be cajoled into declining a therapy at the eventual expense of his or her health, possibly resulting in death. These situations tend to be uncommon, and in the case of therapy, national health insurance would all but eliminate the potential.

APPLICATION TO NATIONAL HEALTH INSURANCE

Now let us examine a few specific privacy-related problems and how any national health insurance plan would likely intensify or abate them. The most favorable result addresses discrimination in obtaining health insurance. If a national plan is implemented, there would be no discrimination *per se*, except perhaps for supplementary policies. The obvious solution to the latter is to make the plan's benefits sufficient to eliminate the necessity for such policies, or at least to a significant degree. True enough, this will make the "premiums" more expensive, yet less than the combination of lesser benefits plus the cost of a supplement.

On the negative ledger, job discrimination is something of a so-called "mixed bag." If the discrimination is based on the costs of health insurance, per se, then the problem would no longer exist. But if the problem is refusing to hire a potential employee because of the effect that a medical condition (or potential condition) might have on job effectiveness, relationships with co-workers, or absenteeism, then we have a major problem, notwithstanding the Americans with Disabilities Act (ADA). Once again, the solution is to restrict access to private data, combined with severe penalties for unauthorized access and misuse.

Of more significance, perhaps, is coercion when it comes to medical services. On the plus side, a national health care plan would virtually eliminate incentives to curtail health care services, especially if each service was be paid for on a fee basis and each hospitalization on a per diem basis (within the minimum-and-maximum range of days for that disease related group or DRG). Still, costs will predictably increase faster than cost-of-living indexes, hence there will be pressure to reduce benefits or otherwise invoke rationing in some form. This potential becomes all the more threatening if the understandable desire to prolong life, even in the face of obviously terminal conditions, is given free reign. For this, we must resort to keeping the plan at arm's length from government meddling.

Lastly, we must consider fraud and malpractice, or more accurately, the detection of likely fraud and malpractice from the mass of data that would accumulate in the computer support systems for any national health insurance plan. The potential to detect these problems is much stronger than commonly believed, and indeed the federal government and most insurance companies use such techniques extensively, at least to detect fraud. The problem, of course, is that overzealous application could lead to so-called "witch-hunts," which in turn could sour providers and perhaps many patients as well. The potential is serious enough to warrant detailed discussion in chapters 12 and 13 respectively. Suffice it to say here that astute governance of the plan is the only practical way of keeping this problem in bounds.

SAFEGUARDS

Security must begin with the technical aspects of collecting and storing data. The reason is that to the extent such aspects are perforated, the supervisory and enforcement requirements are all the greater, no different than, say, dispersing prisoners in a single penitentiary to a dozen sites with no increase in staffing. For this reason, all data collected in a national health care plan should be limited to a mere two levels: regional and national (beyond what individual providers and institutions must maintain), with strict limitations of access even for the national level on regional data. Figure 8 illustrates the simplest possible paradigm.

The second most important safeguard is to enact severe penalties for misuse of data or even unauthorized access. Here again, detection is facilitated by severely limiting the number of databases or more accurately the segments of a singular database, and concurrently restricting the number of people with access. Actually, both the Social Security Administration and the Internal Revenue Service are not unfamiliar with unauthorized access to their respective databases, and accordingly severe enforcement provisions are provided.

The third, and arguably the most important safeguard is to keep arm's length between the database and the government, if only because it would be too tempting for the latter to abuse the data "in the interests of public health." We are only too familiar with the abuses spawned under the supposed justification of "national security."

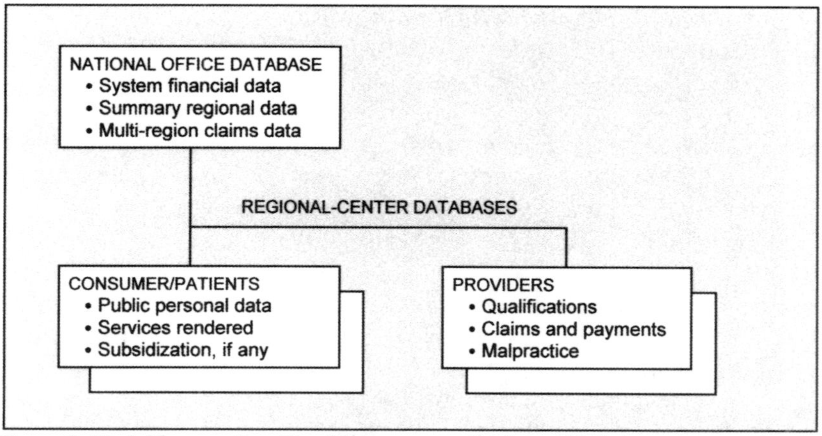

Figure 8. Model for a national health insurance database. *While it may seem naive that the database to support a national health insurance plan could be as simple as depicted here, in point of fact current automation technology makes it entirely possible.*

POTENTIAL FOR A CORE NATIONAL DATABASE

It is fairly obvious that any effective national health insurance plan would require a database that held data on virtually every citizen and legal alien in the United States. Understandably this worries many observers, notwithstanding any security measures put in place to guard against unauthorized access and abuse thereof. But in point of fact at least seven national databases already exist, some of which constitute multiple, overlapping databases. They include:

- ***Social Security.*** This database includes virtually every U.S. citizen from shortly after birth, and most resident aliens.

- ***Internal Revenue Service.*** This includes better than 97 percent of citizens over the age of 16, and aliens who earn income, plus all corporations and businesses.

- ***Credit reporting agencies.*** This includes better than 95 percent of all citizens over 18 years of age. Actually, there are at least three independent databases.

- ***Marketing databases.*** These databases probably include even a higher percentage of citizens. While not every person has credit, everyone buys goods.

• ***Internet, telephone and locator directories.*** These exist whether the number is listed, unpublished, or unlisted, and probably cover 97 percent of households, as well as all businesses.

• ***Conduct and behavior-oriented databases.*** These are not well publicized but exist they do and are surreptitiously consulted by numerous businesses and agencies. For the most part, data is culled from public records.[3]

• ***Decennial census records.*** The attempt is 100 percent coverage, but obviously the data rapidly loses accuracy in the interim decades. But what do we mean by a national *core* database? Simply this: a singular database containing only basic *public* information on each citizen and alien (whether resident or temporary). Some of the data would be mandatory, i.e., name, date of birth, citizenship status, gender, jurisdiction of domicile, etc. Other data would be optional at the election of the person, *e.g.*, addresses and telephone numbers. All other databases which simply use this "front end" data for their own records, either by continually updated copies or by direct access. The public would have open access to any and all data on the core database, but none of the appendant databases. Figure 9 outlines the concept schematically.

A national core database would offer at least three major advantages in general:

• ***Elimination of overlapping and conflicting databases.*** This is prima facie and a vast money-saver.

• ***Assistance in anti-terrorism, and for that matter, all bona fide law enforcement.*** This is self-explanatory, and if a supplementary record included a digital image of the individual, it would facilitate reduction of so-called identity theft.

• ***Elimination of a separate decennial census.*** The "census" would always be current, though it is understood additional data may have to be collected, some on a total survey basis, the balance by sampling.

With respect to national health insurance, perhaps the primary advantage would be the assurance that each individual paid their premiums or had them paid for them. In turn, this would facilitate determination of

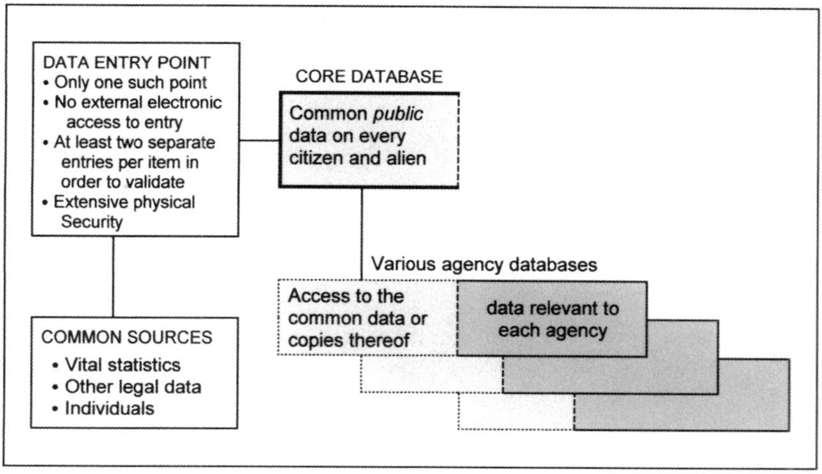

Figure 9. Model for a core national data base. *The idea behind a core national database is to eliminate inconsistencies and overlaps among many other databases. It would eliminate numerous record-keeping problems that would be faced by any national health insurance plan. But only the core data would be accessible by the public at large.*

eligibility for subsidization, both in terms of the premiums and co-payment assistance.

On the other hand, any national core database would also evoke several disadvantages, chief among them a sense of "big brother," notwithstanding that many such databases already exist. Second, the cost of maintaining the core database could excessively tax the health insurance program, should that cost be satellited entirely on the plan, which it should not, as it would service many other agencies.

Still, such a database could be used to expand the new national "do not call" registry aimed at telemarketers. Simply put, every individual could elect to indicate a no-junk-mail-or-telemarketing calls (if they chose to list their address and/or telephone number). An exception field could be made for charities in which at least 90 percent of the proceeds were applied directly to the work of the charity. Everyone knows that the Postal Service uses the profits, as it were, of first class mail to subsidize advertising mail. It is understandable that we have to pay to have garbage removed. Why do we have to pay to receive it?

The third problem concerns the witness protection program, wherein certain individuals are given new identities, complete with new Social Security numbers. Unfortunately, if the core database were made fully public, anyone can screen the entire database to detect "new" Social

Security numbers coupled with a date of birth that in effect tells the user that said person is in the witness protection program. There may be ingenious ways to bypass this problem, but they all involve a cumbersome apparatus.

Chapter 12

Fraud

Our greatest error is that we suppose mankind more honest than they are.

-Alexander Hamilton

FRAUD HAS MANY definitions, yet they all seem to be minor variations of the long-standing definition found in *Black's Law Dictionary*, to wit: "An intentional perversion of truth for the purpose of inducing another in reliance upon it to part with some valuable thing belonging to him or to surrender a legal right."[1] Hence, when a provider files a claim on an insurance company or Medicare for a service not rendered, it is fraud pure and simple.

The major point here is that fraud has little to do with medical professionalism, and virtually no one in the health care field offers any justification for it. Yet it is ubiquitous and a major cost factor. Indeed, the loss being in excess of fifty billion dollars annually, its elimination could fund most all presently unmet health care needs at the present level of funding. In this chapter, then, we briefly measure the extent of fraud in medical insurance, and for that matter, in the United States in general, and what can be done to virtually eliminate all but the most minor instances of it under a national health insurance plan.

EXTENT AND FORMS OF FRAUD

Despite various notions that "mankind is basically good," fraud is rampant, which also suggests massive public indifference if not toleration, or at least an unwillingness of the government to make more of a dent in it than occurs. The following items provide some indication of the magnitude:

- ***Federal income tax fraud.*** The estimated amount of *fraudulently* unpaid income tax is on the order of $216 billion. Annually.[2] To be sure, much of this tax is based on illegal activities, but that does not make it any the less due and payable. Recall that Alphonse Capone was incarcerated on income tax evasion charges sixty-four years ago.

• ***Consumer insurance fraud.*** Consumers and business file fraudulent claims in the amount of $27.6 billion annually.[3] Of that amount, $12.3 billion is attributed to false private automobile claims; $1.8 billion, phony homeowners policy claims; and most of the balance—$12 billion of it—from various businesses and commercial enterprises. Interestingly, businesses pay only 10 percent of the total federal taxes, but are guilty of nearly half of the fraudulent insurance claims.

In the field of health care fraud, the current estimate is in excess of $100 billion annually, about one-tenth of total health care spending.[4] What makes the picture even more drastic is the fact that the Federal Bureau of Investigation now assigns more than 500 agents to investigate this category of fraud, and is currently investigating more than 3000 cases.[5] In any event, we find at least three forms on the part of providers, and several more on the part of consumers and patients.

• ***Billing for services not rendered, including padding.*** This is by far the most common form. In the case of a per diem and/or per dysfunction reimbursement system for hospitals, the potential for fraudulent overcharges would be eliminated, but individual providers could still attempt to milk the system. Unfortunately, even if outright fraud is all but eliminated, the magnitude of unnecessary services would likely increase.

• ***Intentionally leading a patient to accept a medical service for which there is no need or justification.*** This, too, is fraud by definition, notwithstanding that the service is provided. It is no different than, say, an automobile shop "persuading" a customer that his or her car engine needs an overhaul when in fact it merely needs a tune-up. That is to say, the service may be performed, and it may even be performed competently, but the customer is still out the money for unneeded services. On the other hand, and unlike billing for goods and services not rendered, anything less than a clear-cut, unmistakable lack of necessity shifts the case into malpractice, if at all.

• ***Attempting to collect excess charges from a patient despite legal prohibition.*** This, too, is fraud because the patient is not obliged to pay such charges. This occurs primarily in Medicare, and to a lesser extent in the military plan known as TriCare. The fraud arises from the assumption that perhaps many patients will pay or at least attempt to pay whatever they are billed. Unfortunately, research data on this form is weak, despite perhaps a majority of the population having experienced it at one time or another.

This is not to say that consumers are all that innocent. Patients exercise fraud in at least two ways, omitting the rare case of a patient directly filing a claim for insurance benefits that were not received:

• ***Portraying a greater state of indigence than is the case.*** This often occurs in the Medicaid program and Veterans Administration, of which a variation is conceal assets in order to qualify.

• ***Claiming non-existent symptoms for the purpose of obtaining unnecessary medical services or prescriptions, covered by insurance.*** Although this is a kind of consumer parallel to medical malpractice, it nevertheless constitutes fraud, no less so than a provider who persuades a patient to accept a totally unnecessary service. It costs the system money just the same.

EASE OF DETECTION IN CENTRALIZED SYSTEMS

The great problem in reducing fraud, aside from public indifference, is the difficulty of detecting it. Fortunately, in centralized fiduciary systems detection is much easier, which would be the case in any national health insurance plan. Moreover, public indifference could be easily bypassed. This is somewhat analogous to banks. Banks are still robbed because there are so many of them and it is therefore all but impossible to prevent it, though modern technology has vastly improved subsequent apprehension and prosecution. But when it comes to gold, the entire federal reserves are maintained in exactly one location—Fort Knox. That facility is so secure that as far as is known no one has every seriously contemplated breaking in. Not even the fictional Blofeld in Ian Fleming's *Goldfinger* attempted to rob it; only to contaminate the gold with radiation.

To be sure, a computer system hardly offers the protection of Fort Knox, witness the prevalence of successful hackers and countless "viruses." But what such systems may lack in preventive measures they more than compensate with ease of detection after the fact. After all, once detected and prosecuted, the funds are usually recovered and the culprit incarcerated or at least identified as a felon.

The process of detection is a form of decision support system, itself an outgrowth of what is wishfully called "artificial intelligence." There is nothing magic here. Rather, such systems identify the anomalies that are almost certain to crop up in fraud, precisely because fraudulent claims are by their very nature out of the ordinary. Perhaps the most prevalent use of these detection systems occurs with the Internal Revenue Service (IRS), which subjects every return to computer-based analysis. This doesn't mean that every fraudulent return is detected, or that every return so earmarked is actually fraudulent. But the batting average is exceptionally high.

The problem here is that the indifference is manifested in Congress in the form of voter-pleasing in an attempt to secure re-election, manifested by reducing funds hence the number of IRS agents. The same is not true of many commercial insurance companies, who must collectively deal with millions of fraudulent and/or padded claims annually. Hence, the application to health care insurance is merely a matter of applying existing technology to a more comprehensive database. The ultimate idea is simple: If every sustained attempt at fraud is bound to be caught, a lot fewer providers will attempt it.

Still, if this proves insufficient, there remains the informant route, which is much more prevalent than commonly perceived. Indeed, the majority of criminal cases are brought to trial by way of informants, and the Internal Revenue Service has relied on this practice to a significant extent to nab tax cheats. Granted, the practice has a tendency to weaken trust, but keep in mind that its use would be limited to criminal fraud, not malpractice.

Lastly, the matter of penalties must be considered. If we acknowledge that fraud above certain misdemeanor threshold values constitutes a felony, it would be easy enough for any national health insurance plan to deny all future reimbursement to any physician or other provider who is found guilty of fraud or to any hospital that keeps such a provider on their medical staff.

Chapter 13
Malpractice

Against stupidity the gods themselves rail in vain.

– J. F. C. Schiller

UNLIKE FRAUD, MALPRACTICE encompasses a wide range of behaviors, from not using procedure mildly supported by research findings to the intentional killing of a patient. To be sure, these extremes are not normally considered malpractice. The first is a matter of professional judgment and not normally actionable in civil court. The second is a capital felony and is inevitably tried in a criminal court, though the next of kin can also sue for damages. For all between, the issue is not of criminality but incompetence and lack of sound professional judgment.

SITUATION

In its own right, a national health insurance plan is not likely to make much of a dent in malpractice *per se*. The one possibility is that the massed, integrated databases could facilitate detection of potential malpractice in some cases, and as a corollary, the malpractice "records" of physicians and other providers could be listed on another database and made public. Actually, the latter is already in existence—the National Practitioner Data Base—but to date the public does not have access to it.[1] And as mentioned in a previous chapter, physicians have retaliated after a fashion by using a privately operated national database—*CourtScan*—that tracks malpractice cases filed by patients. The objective is to avoid them for all but emergency care.

In all, we have here a potentially destabilizing problem if for no other reason that physicians and their various associations, as in all other professions, are reluctant to discipline their members for all but the most malignant practices. Hence, we need to examine the scope of the problem and lay down some guidelines to both reduce malpractice somewhat and at the same time to keep the procedures from getting out of hand.

Actually, this process is already underway in a few states, most notably Massachusetts and Florida, both of which offer toll-free numbers and web-sites for consumers to obtain a fairly comprehensive report on any doctor licensed to practice medicine in their respective jurisdictions.[2]

FORMS OF MALPRACTICE

Although there is no agreement on categorization of malpractice, the vast majority of cases short of the extremes can be lumped under four categories:

- ***Outright incompetence.*** This is where the physician or other provider simply does not have sufficient knowledge and/or skill to consistently practice well in his or her field of specialization. The Roman Catholic Church calls this invincible ignorance. It cannot be overcome, at least not by the parameters by which medicine normally operates.

- ***Avoidable situational shortcomings.*** A family practitioner would be guilty of severe malpractice if he or she attempted neurosurgery, though that same provider could be the epitome of family practice. Alternatively, an otherwise competent physician or provider can take on more cases under less than emergency circumstances, that in turn significantly increases the risk of failure or at least reduces the chance of success. The adjective *avoidable* is crucial; we are not talking about so-called "good Samaritan" cases, which moreover are protected by law in every state of the Union.

- ***Devolution of technology.*** This means a failure to use newer procedures or other therapies that have been reasonably established as more effective, or likely to be more effective, in a specific case than the procedure that was used. There is no clear dividing line between research findings and recommendations that should be considered optional, and those that approach conservative medicine, but the devolution from one to the other is itself recognized in the literature.

- ***Failure to sustain life in what is presumed to be an end-of-life case.*** This is a minefield, and is especially aggravating in the absence of a so-called "living will" or where the medical condition at issue is known to generate a wide range of survival times.

CORRECTIVE MEASURES

It would not be the intent of a national health insurance plan to reduce malpractice. Still, it would be a tempting target for cost cutters. The primary reason is the high cost of malpractice insurance which doubled in cost in late 2001 and which is passed on to the consumer via higher fees for service. The secondary reason is that malpractice usually requires corrective treatment, or that failing, at least the necessary treatment to resolve the medical condition. In so doing, the following factors apply:

- Perhaps the biggest problem is the unwillingness of physicians to discipline errant members in all but the most flagrant cases. Yet any attempt to *directly* bulldoze this failing of human nature will likely do more damage than good, if for no other reason than the "witch-hunt" syndrome.

- The actual cases of malpractice pursued in court are a matter of public record.

- Determination of malpractice outside of a courtroom, even if accurate, does not normally result in disciplinary action, at least not in the absence of numerous complaints against the same individual within a relatively short time.

- Malpractice on the part of hospitals or staff thereof does not lend itself to significant disciplinary action short of effectively closing down that hospital by way of rescinding its accreditation.

- Patterns of malpractice are not as easily detected from data as patterns of fraud, although the combination of records, complaints, and court cases would enable the managers of the plan to do so.

- One linchpin of a good plan is to maintain professionalism and to end the degrading treatment of professionals by "managed care" clerks.

Thus there are two possible approaches:

- Long-term denial of reimbursement to any provider who crossed certain thresholds of court cases resolved in favor of plaintiffs, say more than two such cases in a period of three years; three cases in five years; and four cases in ten years.

- Widely disseminated summary of court cases and disciplinary actions taken against physicians, readily available to consumers.

In any case, it is best to leave the resolution to professionals, overseen by other authorities only in the case of culpable negligence.

* * * * *

There is also another way to approach the accelerating costs of malpractice insurance, and that is for the medical profession to incorporate or otherwise oversee the creation of its own insurance firm, financially seeded by first-year premiums from all practicing physicians who elect to be covered by its policies. This approach, of course, would be impractical to implement under the present non-system of health care insurance. But it would be more than feasible under national health care insurance because the vast majority of physicians would derive their income from a single source and thus be de facto unified into a single entity.

The primary rationale is that a physician-based malpractice insurance company would almost decimate current premiums, reducing them on average to less than a third of existing rates. Why? First, there would be no need to make any profit on the insurance business, per se. Second, there would be a very strong motivation to contest ludicrous proposed settlements. (The majority of malpractice suits are settled out of court, as are virtually all types of tort cases.) Commercial insurance companies tend to simply pass on the costs to physicians. By contrast, a physician-based company would seek more reasonable thresholds. Third, this approach would operate indirectly to reduce malpractice and rid the profession of its most incompetent practitioners.

That third reason would come about by pegging annual premiums to malpractice settlements incurred by each member, at least in proportion to appropriate time frames and known differences in inherent susceptibility to malpractice among medical specialities. That is to say, the most incompetent practitioners would sooner or later realize that the cost of their policy would devour far too much of their entire income, hence they would cease practicing. Fee schedules would not be adjusted for individuals to compensate for higher insurance premiums, and commercial premiums, if available, would arguably be even higher.

This also has the additional benefit of eliminating the need for competent physicians to "blow the whistle" on their errant colleagues, or otherwise being perceived to be on a "witch hunt." Neurosurgery is not something that is self-taught; cooking one's own goose is. Or as Benjamin Franklin once wrote: "Experience runs an expensive school, but fools will learn in no other, and scarcely in that one."

For the sake of illustration, then, let us say that 500,000 physicians participate in the plan, and pay an average initial annual premium of $30,000, an absolute bargain compared to current commercial rates. That would result in a $15 billion pool of money, which is more than the sum total of all malpractice awards in a year, many of which are settled at too high an amount.

On the other hand, a malpractice insurance firm operated under the aegis of physicians would not prove to be a means of further increasing physician income beyond the one-time reduction of unconscionable increases to commercial premiums. Under any national health insurance plan, reimbursable fees would be held to what is reasonable, not as low as scraping-the-bottom-of-the-barrel Medicare schedules but not Midas-level either. In short, the malpractice-insurance-premium situation has become something of a micro crisis within a macro crisis, and it must be resolved with the same degree of reasonableness as the superintending problem.

PART V
POLITY

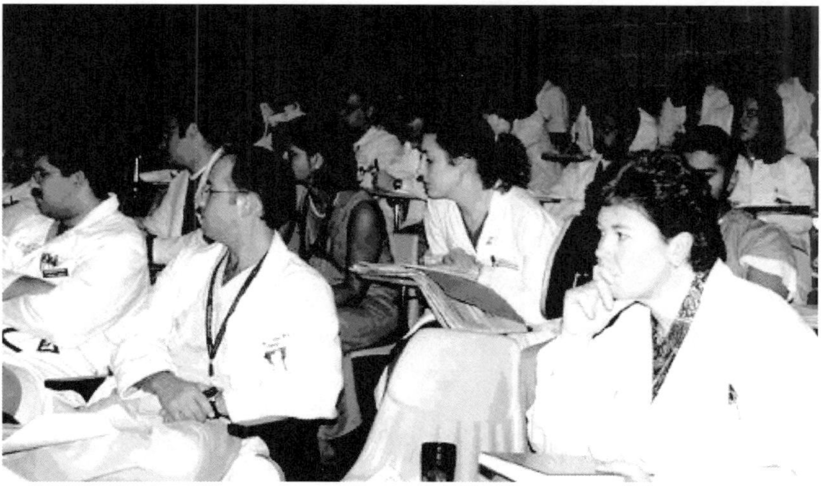

Courtesy: University of New Jersey Medical School.

THE SCENE IS familiar to all physicians—making grand rounds in medical school and residency programs. This is one of the hallmarks of the medical profession: passing on the torch of knowledge and expertise to the next generation, and with it a demand for even more competence. Still, the growing problem of cost-based inaccessibility may soon cause the polity to substitute "efficiency" for professionalism. Only the profession of medicine itself can avoid that serious mistake.

Chapter 14
Sclerosis

Dost thou not know, my son, with how little wisdom the world is governed?

– Bengt Oxenstierna, 1680

A NATIONAL HEALTH insurance plan can only be developed and operated under the aegis of the federal government. All other alternatives are impractical, to say the least. To begin with, the plan would absorb Medicare, Medicaid, the funding of most Veterans Administration health care facilities and probably stateside military hospitals. Premiums or their equivalent must be collected, and subsidies provided for the poor, both in terms of premiums and co-payments. Lastly, costs ultimately must be controlled, and there must be mechanisms to adjust reimbursements in times of economic depression and severe recessions.

By the same token, however, an arm's length relationship between the federal government and the plan and its providers is indispensable and inviolate. This would be the only way the plan could be kept from political manipulation for diverse ends that have little to do with medicine. Or more likely, to keep government officials—at times, mere clerks—from meddling in the professional judgment of physicians and other providers. Or expanding coverage under the best of intentions but with indifference to the cost consequences and eventual ruination of the plan.

This means that the medical profession should take the initiative while openly and honestly negotiating with Congress and the executive branch of the government. That is a tall order, yet the practice of medicine offers an almost unique set of parameters that auger success. First, and from an insurance viewpoint, the plan would offer ultimate compactness, and it would be based largely on the successful Canadian system (adding effective cost controls). Second, the problem of insurance availability is approaching crisis dimensions. Third, medicine is arguably the most prestigious among all professions, and it has the clout to resist government interference should the latter grow too heavy, namely to temporarily cease to provide services except where life is at stake.

In this chapter, then, we focus on the intractable problems of the federal infrastructure. Professional initiative can bypass these problems without causing any Constitutional impasse.

MAGNITUDES AND DEMOGRAPHICS

The Constitution of the United States is one of the most venerable documents of all time. If we assume the first ten amendments—the Bill of Rights—were *de facto* an integral part of the original document, then it is almost startling how little the subsequent eighteen amendments modified the Constitution.[1] Still, conditions have changed which have skewed the numbers, so to speak, and which therefore make the federal mechanics less adaptable to our own times. Five of the most significant changes have been:

- ***Population.*** This has increased nearly a hundred-fold, from 3 to 286 million.

- ***Area.*** In terms of settled land, this has increased about forty-fold, and nearly ten-fold in terms of land owned. Moreover, that land is far more intensely used.

- ***Role of government.*** Albeit subjective in terms of laws passed and the federal budget (adjusted for inflation), this too seems to have grown a hundred-fold. Interestingly, the sum total of federal employees located in Washington, D.C., as late as 1829, was a grand total of 30, and that included the military and Congressional staff.[2]

- ***Federal vs. state jurisdictions.*** As late as 1861, Robert E. Lee was able to renounce his citizenship in the United States in favor of his home state of Virginia, in order to defend the rights of the latter, and be thought a gentleman for it. Bear in mind that General Winfield Scott, chief of staff of the Army at the time, had offered Lee command of the Union army. Today, the idea would be ludicrous, and more to the point, one only need "weigh" the substance and influence of federal laws vs. state laws in any state.

- ***Communications and transportation.*** This, too, is subjective in part, but suffice it to say that the fastest communications and travel in 1789 were by horseback or sailing ship for those on coastlines,

> sending a message to England, and receiving a reply, took two months. Today, image transmission worldwide is instantaneous, and one can travel to any place in the United States in less than eight hours.

Of perhaps more significance is the disproportion of voting strength among the states, combined with the fact that there are fifty of them, almost four times the original thirteen. Every schoolboy knows about the great compromise made during the Constitutional convention in 1787, whereby the less changeable Senate comprised equal representation by states, while the House of Representatives was established proportional to population. That paradigm remains untouched to this day, except for a proportional increase in the total number of representatives. Yet, this fixed rule has created a major problem in effective voting. A mere tenth of the population constitutes a majority vote in the Senate. The reason is that the twenty-five least populated states claim roughly 10 percent of the population.[3] This proportion is actually much lower than one-tenth because a Senator is rarely elected by more than 60 percent of the 55 percent or so of the population that does vote.

ECONOMIC FACTORS

Now let us turn briefly to various aspects of national economics, of which lobbying, campaigning, and the infamous "pork barrel" command the most publicity. For the first seventy-five years of the nation's life, Congress was low budget, lobbying was low key and more often than not aimed at qualitative issues, and there was comparatively little "pork." Today, we have the opposite picture, especially when mere campaigns for re-election to the House of Representatives can cost upwards of several million dollars, sometimes tens of millions. As for pork, the total amount is commonly estimated to be of the order of $18.5 billion, which aside from funding for entitlements and the minimum required to run various departments and programs, amounts to 20 percent or more of the balance, *i.e.*, of the discretionary funds.[4] Of course, the executive branch is not innocent; one only need consider the amount of time presidents spend dunning supporters for campaign funds. But perhaps the worst aspect of this situation is that research now indicates that most votes in Congress are more or less for sale.[5]

Still, the critical item here is the growing welfare state, which does not auger well for a quasi-independent insurance plan that looks to personal responsibility insofar as possible. True enough, much has been written about the reduction of welfare rolls over the past five years, which was achieved by placing limits on the years an individual could collect certain forms of welfare (with exceptions). What is not commonly broadcast is that many of those who were ejected simply became homeless or had to be satellited on private charities (and that was before recessionary times). Moreover, that kind of welfare is but a small fraction of the overall welfare funding at the federal level, which is often called by the euphemism of "income redistribution" or "tax breaks." But have no doubts; it is welfare pure and simple, and it is reaching a trillion dollars a year. The main items:

- ***Earned income tax credit.*** To any person or married couple with one or more children, with a gross income not exceeding $31,951, the federal government grants a non-taxable supplement up to $3888 (for the tax year 2000). In many, perhaps most cases, the amount exceeds tax liability, including Social Security, hence constitutes a true negative income tax. The respective figures for 2001 are $2428 (one child) and $4008 (two or more children).

- ***Income tax rates and deductions.*** To no one's surprise, the poor pay no income tax or only negligible amounts. Indeed, of those who file returns, the lowest 20 percent in taxable income pay only 3/10 tenths of 1 percent of the total personal income tax collected, and this is more than offset by the earned income tax credit.[6]

- ***Social Security benefits and taxability.*** Despite the claim that Social Security benefits are proportional to income, hence to taxes paid in, the benefits are heavily skewed in favor of low income earners. Furthermore, federal income tax is levied on Social Security benefits when total income exceeds certain threshold levels, which creates the situation where in some cases, an individual who paid $2N in Social Security tax over a lifetime may receive a net benefit less than another individual who paid only $N.[7]

- ***Supplementary Security Income.*** This is welfare for nearly seven-million persons, in addition to Social Security benefits (if eligible), in the amount of $29 billion annually.[8]

- ***Food stamps.*** These non-taxable trade-for-food coupons are given to low income earners, in the total amount of $17.7 billion annually.[9]

• ***Various government pensions and related benefits.*** This does not refer to retired military and Civil Service pensions (which are generous), but to pensions such as Veteran's disability. The VA alone provides $46.8 billion worth of programs annually.[10]

Perhaps the extent of this welfare situation is best shown by the benefits that can be paid to a couple who intentionally avoid a legal marriage. If each person has one child, and each earns $12,000 per year (and assuming they claim only the standard deduction), they would each pay $918 in Social Security tax, offset by $2353 each in earned-income tax credits. Thus their combined "take-home" pay on income of $24,000 would be $26,870 (not counting the value of food stamps, for which they would normally be eligible for approximately $1000). But if they were married, their take-home pay on $24,000 would be $22,844, that is, an increase in taxes of $4026. For the tax year 2001, and assuming incomes of $12,300 each, the increase would be $4498 (plus reduced food-stamps, if any).

Actually, we could say that at least 90 percent of the nation's population is on the dole in one form or another, and indeed, 24 percent of the population pays 81 percent of the personal income taxes.[11]

The last item to cover here is what we might call chronic fiscal irresponsibility, of which the Social Security and other trust funds are the prime example. The problem is, those funds do not exist, except on paper. The monies have all been spent, in return for IOU's from the government in addition to the national debt of more than five trillion dollars. These funds, in the case of Social Security, are intended to fund the deficit between collections and benefits estimated to begin in 2009. But in order to use the funds, the government must either further increase the deficit or severely reduce benefits, or both.

To be sure, economics remains "the dismal science," and very few people understand the operation of economic forces, not even on relatively simple matters. Case in point, and one debated *ad nauseam* in *The Washington Post* in 1986: A car dealer that claimed a potential buyer would pay less interest at 11 percent on an auto loan than he could earn at 6 percent in a savings account. The *Post* invited readers to submit explanations, and gave first prize to a long-winded technical explanation centering on future values.

The actual explanation was much simpler. In the savings account the *entire* principle remains in the account for the four years, whereas the auto loan is amortized over the same period, meaning that—in effect—the full loan value was borrowed for roughly two years. Hence two years interest at 11 percent is less than 6 percent interest on the same amount over four years. When this was explained to the *Post* editors in excruciating detail, they did not acknowledge their error, neither to their reading public nor to this writer.[12]

Chapter 15

Factions

We are none of us tolerant in what concerns us deeply and entirely.

– Samuel T. Coleridge

ANY SIGNIFICANT CHANGE in the polity will engender resistance. Voters will likely favor national health insurance, but Congress and the Executive Office will just as likely milk it for objectives that have little to do with the plan itself. In this chapter, we essay some of the special interests that will lobby Congress to mold the plan to their liking.

HOSPITALS

In general, hospitals will welcome national health insurance, The primary reason is that insurance reimbursement has become a game of "robbing Peter to pay Paul," primarily because of the need to provide either free or inadequately reimbursed care. This is especially true of emergency rooms, where all comers must be provided for, at least until the condition underlying the complaint is stabilized. Then, too, these same emergency rooms are often the only provider available for indigent patients with non-emergency conditions.

On the negative side, lower-occupancy hospitals may seek to preserve their "right" to continue providing care. And of more significance, the proprietary hospitals (750 of 5850 or 13 percent) will likely insist on their "right" to continue making a profit. Now if benefits are set to provide adequate reimbursement, and all hospitals are required to take all "comers," it is obvious that the ploy of taking only selected patients in order to maximize profits will be eliminated.

A third problem is the reimbursement for teaching hospitals, which of necessity must be higher, and this can easily be provided for in the reimbursement schema. And a fourth problem concerns the military and

VA hospitals, which need not be severe if the plan is seen primarily as a reimbursement mechanism that is at least as good, and probably much better, than present funding.

HEALTH MAINTENANCE ORGANIZATIONS

Under this plan, the HMO's could continue to operate but only as a variation on group practice. Reimbursement would be on the basis of service rendered and per hospitalization. There would be no per capita annual payments. Hence, those HMO's intent on health care would more than likely support the plan, while those that were more intent on squeezing profits from the capitation payments would not.

INSURANCE COMPANIES

The reactions will vary, albeit primarily negative. This is because virtually all health insurance will be eliminated, and possibly the need for most supplementary insurance. Nor would these firms be needed as administrators of a national plan, at least not if the plan is well designed. The reason is that under the proposal in this book, the vast majority of claims review, marketing, advertising, etc., would be eliminated. The emphasis would be on exception processing and reacting to anomalies that arose from analysis of collective data. Moreover, almost all of this processing would be automated. In short, the idea is to all but eliminate the high costs of claims processing and profits for that matter. Stand by to repel boarders.

EMPLOYERS AND UNIONS

Both employers and unions will strongly endorse national health insurance, especially if it reduces costs or alternatively provides health care for the same cost. The issues will concern the employer's share and what each employee must contribute.

STATE GOVERNMENTS

They will probably welcome the plan because it relieves them of the problems of funding care for the indigent, though whatever funding is currently provided should be redirected into the common "pot" of any national plan. The more serious problem will be in potential loss of jurisdiction with respect to authority for licensure and related matters, and de facto on the matter of regulating health insurance. Although the model stresses the insurance aspects, it is reasonable to assume that pressures will be brought to bear to overrule or bypass various aspects of state responsibilities and prerogatives.

PHARMACEUTICAL MANUFACTURERS

They will oppose the plan to the extent they presume universal coverage may zero in on excess—some would say obscene—profits. Of course, it cannot oppose national health insurance directly. Instead, it will intensify its lobbying of Congress, which has a tendency to sell out to the highest bidder.[1] So it is to that institution we must again turn.

CONGRESS

The perennial problem in Congress is the tendency of the Republican party to sell out to big business, and for the Democratic party to sell out to whomever will vote for them. As shown in table 6, the Democratic party now appeals to so-called minority voters, and quite successfully.

Table 5. Voting by racial/ethnic categories in the year 2000

Category	**Percent**	**Percent voting**			**Index values for the vote**		
		Dem.	**Rep.**	**Other**	**Dem.**	**Rep.**	**Other**
White	80%	42%	54%	4%	33.60	43.20	3.20
African-American	10%	90%	9%	1%	9.00	0.90	0.10
Hispanic	7%	62%	35%	3%	4.34	2.45	0.21
Asian	2%	55%	41%	4%	1.10	0.82	0.08
Other voters	1%	55%	39%	6%	0.55	0.39	0.06
Total	**100%**				**48.59**	**47.76**	**3.65**

Source: U.S. News and World Report, November 20, 2000, p. 40. Data for "other percent voting" was calculated simply by subtracting the two percentages for the major parties from 100%.

In theory, of course, national health insurance should be developed beyond partisan politics. In theory. But once again we need to remind ourselves that such insurance will constitute the single greatest concentration of funds in the nation's history and will prove irresistible to political manipulation. It is therefore imperative that the developers of the plan take this into account, and preferably establish it before the federal government turns headlong into socialism. And that day may not be too far off.

Why? Consider the data above. The lesson is that in order to win the White House in the near-term future, the Republican party must win approximately 60 percent of non-minority voters, especially if the Democratic party succeeds in registering minority voters in proportion to their strength in the general population. That is, in the election year 2000, it took 54 or 55 percent of the non-minority vote to win the election, but once the minority vote gains a bigger percentage of the vote (say 24 percent rather than 17 percent), and continues to vote they way it does, then it will take 60 percent, or more, of the non-minority vote to win.

The point, of course, is that in order to maintain those votes, the Democratic party must promise even more benefits and related government programs. Granted, there is a measure of justice to some of these programs in light of past injustices faced by minorities, yet there is a price to pay when the government goes too far in this direction. It doesn't take the proverbial rocket scientist to estimate what would happen to the costs under a national health care plan if it is not kept at arm's length from presidential contenders and Congress. It is not going too far to say that the way we go about implementing national health insurance will set the stage for the entire polity during the ensuing century.

Chapter 16

Professionalism

The functionaries of every government have propensities to command at will the liberty and property of their constituents.

– Thomas Jefferson

EVERY PROFESSION HAS its paragons. Sometimes they are historical persons, but more often exemplary fictional characters. In the profession of law, it is hard to identify a better example of competence, integrity, and admirable character than Atticus Finch in Harper Lee's *To Kill a Mockingbird.* In the ministry, a character of equal caliber is Raymond Kumalo, the Anglican priest in Alan Paton's *Cry, the Beloved Country*, especially as portrayed in the cinematographic remake starring James Earl Jones.

For medicine, the odds-on favorite is the TV character Marcus Welby, played by Robert Young. Welby was almost too good to be true, yet he was no less believable than the sterling character of George Washington or Robert E. Lee (of whom Harper Lee is a direct descendent). In one memorable scene, Dr. Welby is counseling a young doctor, who is weighing an opportunity to amass a considerable fortune. In the end, Welby makes his case with a singular comment that one must decide between the profession of medicine and fortune hunting.

Unfortunately, even the opportunity to maintain medicine as a profession is rapidly declining, if for no other reason that so-called "managed care" is rampant. In the event of a carelessly developed national health insurance plan—with its predictable vast cost overruns—the situation is bound to grow worse. It is for this reason that medicine must choose between professionalism versus making a financial killing as long as the opportunity remains. After that, physicians would likely be reduced to de facto employees whose judgment is continually put under the microscope by clerical personnel, and their incomes increasingly reduced, far more so than if they took the necessary initiative to do what should be done.

THE AMERICAN MEDICAL ASSOCIATION

The American Medical Association is the only institution capable of taking the initiative with respect to a national health insurance plan. It is the largest and the most prestigious of medical organizations, and its journal is commonly regarded as second only to the *New England Journal of Medicine*. To be sure, the AMA once had the reputation of a reactionary organization, but that is changing, and it would certainly like to regain membership. To this end, it can develop a model that could evolve into the actual plan. More importantly it could become the primary tool to gain support of its membership by direct involvement, and subsequently to win over the many political and business entities essential for implementation of the plan.

The first step would be simple enough, namely, development of a reliable computer model to estimate the costs and benefits of a national plan. This does not mean a sophisticated model with all sorts of high-level statistical formulas but rather a basic model stressing quantities and simple factors. The appendix provides some specifications for such a model, and it may behoove the AMA to have two or three models developed independently and then test them until they all produce essentially the same answers under the same conditions.

The second step would be to "distribute" the model, via the Internet if nothing else, complete with a questionnaire to ascertain how physicians respond to various options. Such a questionnaire might have two sections: (a) a series of objective items that are easily tabulated, primarily on various options that a plan may offer, and (b) a comment section in which there are no limitations to responses.

The third step would be an expansion on the second, namely to expand distribution to relevant organizations and various government agencies, except that by this point the medical profession should have developed a fairly comprehensive plan.

The fourth step would be to create the embryo for the plan's board of trustees, and here it would be appropriate to request Gerald Ford and Jimmy Carter to extend their leadership of the national health initiative to serve as co-chairmen of this working group. Reasons:

- ***Arm's length.*** It is imperative that the insurance plan be kept at arm's length from government meddling, while at the same time recognizing that the plan must operate under the aegis of the federal government. The two former presidents, one a Republican the other a Democrat, have the prestige to achieve this.

• ***Magnitude.*** The plan, and any alternative plans for long-term care and dentistry, would easily exceed a trillion dollars. This would be the largest slice of the national economy, and it would be concentrated in a comparatively few hands.

• ***Setting an example.*** As noted in a previous chapter, and summarized in the closing comment, the concept of non-government infrastructure taking the initiative to develop a federal program is something that could be applied to many other high cost programs. The results could set the domestic tone of government for the foreseeable future.

As for the other three former presidents, Ronald Reagan is no longer well, George Bush's son is the present incumbent of the White House, and Mr. Clinton's record is arguably a disqualifier. Among other matters, he has been barred from practicing before the U.S. Supreme Court. Moreover, it is commonly alleged that his wife Hillary has presidential ambitions and would arguably manipulate Mr. Clinton to that end.

RECAPITULATION OF ISSUES

In this penultimate section we recapitulate the ten most difficult issues that any national health insurance plan must resolve, assuming that no physician in his right mind would ever condone fraud or obvious malpractice, and could hardly oppose a policy that requires all providers to *accurately* inform patients of their options and probabilities of various therapies.

• ***Exclusions and inclusions.*** About 10 percent of the potential coverages will cause the most heated debate, especially abortion.

• ***Sources and collection of premiums.*** The biggest sub-issue will be flat-rate vs. scaled premiums, despite subsidization of the poor.

• ***Subsidization and co-payments, especially with respect to Medicare.*** The biggest problem here will be on significant co-payments to preclude over-use of the system.

• ***Reimbursement schemas.*** Most of these issues are technical in nature, but they are likely to indirectly eliminate HMOs (except perhaps as residual group practices) and proprietary hospitals.

• ***Incorporation of government health care resources, such as Veteran's Administration and stateside military hospitals.*** It is not difficult to imagine the "turf" battles on this score, notwithstanding that the plan addresses funding, not ownership.

• ***Control of hospital beds.*** This is another contentious issue because it crosses legal jurisdictions.

• ***Pharmaceuticals.*** The pharmaceutical manufacturers will likely scramble the largest lobbying effort in history in order to preserve their "right" to soak consumers for unconscionable profits.

• ***Rationing in any form, especially situational rationing.*** It is here that ethical and practical and/or economic conflicts will be most sharply focused.

• ***Governance of the plan, to include processing of apparent malpractice.*** This is crucial, unless doctors would just as soon watch a national health insurance plan devolve into an HMO.

• ***Privacy issues.*** These issues are already at the forefront of public consciousness; national health care insurance can only hone the edge more sharply.

CLOSING THOUGHT

While any initiative taken towards a national health insurance plan must concentrate on issues relevant to financing health care, the fact remains that the effort would be a case study applicable to other endeavors. Among those endeavors might be some kind of reform for the legal profession sufficient to abate the bottomless repertoire of lawyer jokes. Then, too, public education could be improved at least to the point where the majority of high school graduates could read and write at an appropriate level. Certainly, all the billions of dollars showered on public schools by the federal government has not done much in the way of improvement, while the record on public schools run by contract is a mixed bag at best.

The list of potential applications could go at considerable length, but perhaps the better course would be to remind ourselves of something

Plutarch wrote in his biographical sketch of Agis:

> For it may happen to the commonwealth, as to the serpent in the fable, whose tail rising in rebellion against the head, complained, as of a great grievance, that it was always forced to follow, and required that it should be permitted by turns to lead the way. And taking the command accordingly, it soon inflicted, by its senseless courses, mischiefs in abundance upon itself, while the head was torn and lacerated with following, contrary to nature, a guide that was deaf and blind. And such we see to have been the lot of many, who, submitting to be guided by the inclinations of an uninformed and unreasoning multitude, could neither stop, nor recover themselves out of the confusion.[1]

Now, the former, long-term editor of the *Journal of the American Medical Association*—George Lundberg—recently concluded that too much greed has permeated the medical profession.[2] Perhaps so, but to date that supposed shortcoming does not remotely match the massive greed evinced in much of American business. I mean, what doctor is on a par with Enron, WorldCom, and at least twenty other major corporations of equivalent ilk? Or with AgraCom, which knowingly shipped tainted chicken to the United States (and several other countries), and after that fowl had been condemned by South Korea? Indeed, this greed is so vast that even Ralph Nader was stunned by its magnitude.[3]

And what is the significance for medicine? At one time, the ballast of American polity was its substantial middle class population. But that was before the middle class began to shrink in proportion *and* the federal government assumed an ever increasing control over people's lives. To the point where it now includes several million part-time "spies" attempting to ferret out any activity that remotely smells of terrorism. Suffice it say that the potential evil of this program was sufficient for the U. S. Postal Service to reject any participation in it. Fortunately, the medical profession has the potential to evolve into a new ballast, not only because of its inherent professionalism but also because it significantly touches the lives of virtually every citizen. Stay tuned.

Appendix

Analytical Computer Model

THIS APPENDIX DESCRIBES a computer-based model by which various options and assumptions can be tested in terms of predictable costs and benefits. The model, or more accurately the development of the model, also offers an indirect benefit in that it all but forces proponents of national health insurance to come to grips with the complex qualitative relationships among the many elements that perforce operate in any such plan.

Preliminaries. Assuming that a computer model for planning and development is essential, three other points should be noted:

- ***Development tool.*** The model itself should be capable of expansion from a planning tool into a development tool for preparation of the relevant legislation.

- ***Avoidance of sophisticated statistical formulas.*** The model should operate as close as practical to actual processing, which means pure arithmetic computations and avoidance of statistical estimations. The sole and obvious exception is to use averaging or mean data based on experience, and even at that, factors and indices would enable the user to display computations within likely ranges.

- ***Three independently developed programs.*** Because models are easy to program with today's program generator software, it would be useful to develop at least three different models independently, that is, without collaboration on the part of the programmers. In this way, results using the same input data and factors can be concurrently tested until consistency is obtained. After that, the final selection would likely be based on qualitative criteria, such as clarity of displays and so forth.

Techniques. Computers today compute at a minimum rate of two billion steps a second (with supercomputers running at a trillion steps per second or higher), and operating memory is sufficiently large to hold all necessary data in the program itself, thus reducing processing time of complex runs to a second or so. This also further simplifies the programming, as it is not necessary to prepare separate data files and the associated fetch routines.

- ***Manual preparation.*** Because the quantitative relationship among all the relevant factors or elements is so complex, it would behoove the developers to first prepare extensive charts depicting these relationships. In this way, the three development teams would start out on the same sheet of music.

- ***Use of computer-assisted programming.*** These programming tools, such as *VisualBasic*, are so versatile that only a two-man team is required to program each version of the model: the programmer and another who person immersed in the health insurance process and its data.

Structure and expandability. The driver is the executive control of the program, as it is in virtually all programs, and is more or less "invisible" to the user, except perhaps for an introductory screen. The program itself requires six sub-programs: (1) main menu, (2) data, (3) factors and indexes, (4) algorithms, (5) displays, printing, and archival "files," and (6) networking protocols. This structure is depicted in figure 10.

Menu and reports/displays. These two functions (not to be confused with a generic form of subprogram called a function) will occupy separate subprograms for technical reasons. And as an option, the menu subprogram could be incorporated into, or be directly called by the driver, which would in turn control all other processing. Still, from a purely logical viewpoint, they must be considered together because all menu choices result in either a display of computational results or in another display permitting the user to change the value of factors, etc.

- ***Menu tiers.*** The primary (main) menu simply prompts the user for the type of processing he or she wants the program to execute, e.g., a computation, change of factor, *temporary* change or addition of data, etc. The next tier prompts for specific processing, which

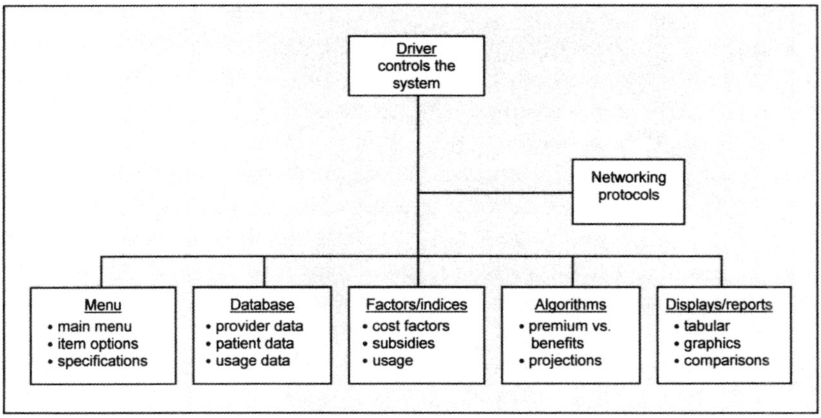

Figure 10. Computer-model structure. *The structure of the model needs at least six subprograms. Each of them should be programmed with the idea of adding many routines as experience dictates, and better yet, permit users to add additional computations without changes to the base algorithms.*

then leads to a third-tier input display (unless the option elected requires no further specifications). Note that experience may suggest making temporary changes and additions permanent, and if so, this should be left to the programmer. Otherwise, the tens of thousands of copies downloaded from Internet distribution would collectively go bananas.

• ***Generic computational displays.*** These outputs should include a summary of the data used, the factors applied, the parameters (if any) selected or entered by the user, and, if the display is complex, the ability to click any field to see a secondary display of more detailed data.

• ***Generic graphic displays.*** These should be an option on any output display that involves a range of answers depending on user-selected options.

• ***Computational differences displays.*** This is a special display that compares the results of two or more compatible computations, which therefore requires a menu display of the N most recent computations.

Database and factors. Although the database and factors are separate sub-programs, they are strongly linked, for example, each item noted below is subject to factoring:

• ***Demographic/population data.*** This will be the most complex part of the program. The reasons are four-fold. The data: (a) is constantly changing, (b) must be divided into regions, complete with cost-indices, (c) broken down by age groups, and (d) annotated for regional variations in medical requirements.

• ***Dysfunction data.*** This is a more-or-less complete run-down on all medical dysfunctions and conditions, and their prevalence by age group and gender.

• ***Provider data.*** Hospitals, physicians, and all other providers, including those who have any chance whatsoever of being included in the benefits package.

• ***Costs.*** This pertains to the two previous items and must be correctly linked.

• ***Sources of funding.*** This, too, is complex, as it must be based on the entire employment paradigm, as well as the retired segment of the population.

Additionally, we have the special case of subsidization parameters, which neatly fall into both data and factors categories. They include cutoff incomes and scaled percentages. Yet fundamentally they are factors, which should operate against demographic, income, and usage data.

Processing and algorithms. Discussion of the comparatively simple algorithms required, or more accurately, the relevant sequences of basic algorithms.

• ***Generic algorithm.*** The most common computation is likely to be a comparison of total costs (exclusive of un-subsidized co-payments) versus total income/premiums, to include a projection over the next three-to-five years by applying various factors. Most of the other computations will likely be a variation on this, or alternatively, a subset of it.

• ***User-specified algorithms.*** This feature will let the user select from types of data, then enter his or her own formula or equation probably by selection from a series of menu-lists, with the program itself generating the relevant algorithm.

End-Notes

1. ***Argument***

1. This information is available on numerous web-sites, for example: <www.pbs.org/criticalcondition/program>. However, the definition of "under-insured" (in contrast to uninsured) is not standard, hence the data varies considerably by source.

2. "Table 3: National Health Expenditures by Source of Funds," Centers for Medicare and Medicaid (formerly Health Care Finance Administration) <www.hcfa.gov>.

2. ***Facts***

1. "Table 108: Hospitals, beds, and occupancy rates," Centers for Disease Control, National Center for Health Statistics, <www.cdc.gov/nchs/products/pubd/hus/tables/2001/01hus108.pdf>.

2. *Ibid.*

3. "Table 12: Median Unadjusted Income of Physicians by years in Practice—1998," American Medical Association, <www.ama-assn.org/ama/pub/article/171-207>.

4. *The New York Times* February 4, 1992, p. A10; Associated Press, October 10, 1990. "Private health insurance far less efficient, more wasteful than Medicare."

5. "Pushing drugs to doctors," *Consumer Reports*, February 1992, pp. 87–94; and "Miracle drugs or media drugs," *Consumer Reports*, March 1992, pp. 142–146.

6. This type of information is exceptionally difficult to pin down to precise numbers because what is "unnecessary" is in large part a medical judgment, and many physicians admitted ordering procedures more to

protect themselves from malpractice suits rather than obvious medical necessity. Furthermore, many unnecessary visits are ordered by physicians as, in effect, a fraudulent practice. Among the many web-sites to check is: <www.os.dhhs.gov/org/oei/whatsnew.htm>.

3. *Undercurrents*

1. This exceptionally rare case involved an anencephalic birth that survived for more than a year (on machines) in Fairfax Hospital, Fairfax, Virginia. The mother wanted to keep the baby alive for as long as possible, but the chairman of the Ethics Committee, Boston University School of Medicine, said: "Technology has the life, not the patient." More to the point, only one ethicist could be found to side with the mother, namely Dr. Robert M. Veatch, Kennedy Institute of Ethics, Georgetown University (a Jesuit institution). At that, Dr. Veatch admitted there was no reason from a medical standpoint for prolonging the life of the organism; only that the mother had the right to make such a choice. *The New York Times,* September 24, 1993, p. A10.

2. Christopher Hogen, et al, "Medical beneficiaries' cost of care in the last year of life," *Health Affairs*, July 2001, pp. 108–195.

4. *Issues*

1. For example, the deductible on a hospital stay was $792 in 2001. There is also an annual deductible under Part B, and then Medicare pays only 80 percent of a physician's fee, to which most physicians tack on another 15 percent.

5. *Systems*

1. Patrick Ryan, "Get rid of the people, and the system runs fine," *Smithsonian,* September, 1977, p. 40.

2. This was the finding of a General Accounting Office report written in July 1993. Ninety percent of claims (at the time) were processed by computer programs; the remaining 10 percent being kicked out to claim reviewers with no medical background and, on average, only a high school diploma. Furthermore, in southern California and in South Carolina, these clerks reviewed an average of 400 claims a day, roughly 72 seconds per claim (assuming they worked eight hours a day without any breaks of any kind).

6. *Mechanics*

1. For example, see "Check out how home prices across USA compare," *USA Today*, July 30, 2001, p. 6B. For a four-bedroom, two-bath, 2,200-square-foot home, prices ranged from $136,050 in Columbus, Georgia; to $1,225,000 in Palo Alto, California, the larger being 900 percent of the lesser.

7. *Governance*

1. In the world of business and government, money in the form of currency has all but evaporated, replaced by ciphers in computer databases. Money is no longer transferred; instead the sending element merely reduces the quantity recorded in the record or file at issue, and the receiving element then increases the corresponding record or file by a like amount (reduced in many instances by a transfer fee). Hence, the question of direct payments to providers from the central accounts of a national health care plan versus prior distribution to regional offices is nearly moot. The regional accounts can be simply "earmarked" in the national account, or they can be transferred electronically to separate accounts. The approach adopted will more than likely be based on legal and technical considerations.

8. *Mainstream*

1. Charles B. Clayman, MD, ed., *The American Medical Association Encyclopedia of Medicine* (New York, Random House, 1989), pp. 270, 755.

2. *See* table 1 in chapter 2 (Centers for Medicare and Medicaid/ HFCA data).

3. *Ibid.*

9. *Periphery*

1. John L. Allen, Jr., *Cardinal Ratzinger: The Vatican's Enforcer of the Faith* (New York: Continuum, 2000), pp. 188-189. Apparently, Cardinal Ratzinger persuaded Pope John Paul II not to declare the Church's dictum against birth control as infallible.

2. *The American Medical Association Encyclopedia of Medicine*, pp. 436, 438.

10. *Psychiatry*

1. John O'Brian, "County defends splitting of Tot-Mom," *Post Standard* (Syracuse), January 18, 1992. I discussed this case with the city editor on February 26, 1993. For additional information on the Kafkaesque nightmare that followed, go to <www.google.com>, enter "denise perrigo syracuse" (without the quotation marks), then visit the first two sites. Among other things, when Mrs. Perrigo took her baby's temperature rectally (the normal procedure in the situation), the county welfare agency charged her with sexual abuse of a child for inserting a foreign object in her baby's rectum.

2. *The American Medical Association Encyclopedia of Medicine*, p. 639.

3. Franz G. Alexander and Sheldon T. Selesnick, *The History of Psychiatry* (New York: Harper & Row, 1966), p. 14.

11. *Privacy*

1. There have been many articles on this subject over the past ten years. For example, *see* Geoffrey Cowley, "Flunk the gene test and lose your insurance," *Newsweek*, December 23, 1996, pp.48–50; and Kim Clark and Josh Fischman, "Out in the Cold," *U.S. News and World Report*, November 12, 2001, pp. 53–65.

2.See "Will Doctors Pay to Know the Names of Malpractice-Prone Patients?" *The Lightning Hypertext of Disease* <www.pathinfo.com/cgi-bin/in.cgi.tx=courtscan>. In its database, this service has more than 802,000 lawsuits (since 1982) filed with the Court of Common Pleas in Pennsylvania. However, attempts to develop parallels in such cities as Detroit, Los Angeles, and Chicago have not been successful.

3. Perhaps the best way to demonstrate the existence of these databases is to quote from a brochure from one of the most reputable companies in the United States, namely Teachers Insurance and Annuity Association (and its sister company College Retirement Equities Fund):

> As part of our routine procedure, we may request that an investigative consumer report be prepared. Such reports typically include information as to identity, general reputation, personal characteristic and mode of living. This information is usually obtained through confidential conversations with neighbors, friends and other acquaintances. . . . This is simply a standard precautionary measure to help assure fair and equitable treatment for everyone concerned. . . . In some situations, and in compliance with applicable laws, we may disclose items of information to third parties.

12. *Fraud*

1. *Black's Law Dictionary*, sixth edition (St. Paul, Minnesota: West Publishing Company, 1990), p. 660.

2. *Congressional Statement on Health-Care Fraud*. Federal Bureau of Investigation. <www.fbi.gov/congress/congress00>. This is part of the annual report on high risk issues within the federal government.

3. *High Risk Series*. The United States General Accounting Office. *See* series six of this annual report of the General Accounting Office (GAO) on high-risk matters. <www.gao.gov/highrisk/hr97002.txt>.

4. "Criminal Fraud Cases." Federal Bureau of Investigation, Health-Care Fraud Unit <www.fbi.gov/hq/cid/fc/hcf/about/hcf_about.htm>. The estimate is just shy of 10 percent of the total spending for health care, which has reached $1.2 trillion.

5. *Ibid.*

13. *Malpractice*

1. *National Practitioner Data Bank*, <www.npdb-hipdb.com>.

2. Christopher J. Gearon, "Unmasking unsafe doctors," *AARP Bulletin*, December 2001, pp. 19–20. Keep in mind that this publication is read by roughly forty million people monthly, probably the most widely read publication in the country.

14. ***Sclerosis***

1. For example, *see* David E. Kyvig, *Explicit and Authentic Acts: Amending the U.S. Constitution 1776–1995* (Kansas City, Kansas: University Press of Kansas, 1996). Of the eighteen amendments enacted since the Bill of Rights, two canceled out each other (prohibition). Most others concern voting rights, election/term-of-office mechanics, and succession in office.

2. Lawrence M. Friedman, *American Law: An Introduction*, revised edition (New York: W.W. Norton, 1998), pp. 131–133.

3. The computation is made by adding populations of the 25 least populous states, which is roughly ten percent of the entire U.S. population but which elects half of the U.S. Senators.

4. "Pork Barrel Spending Grows," *The Waste Basket*, 6:8, (16 March 2001). Taxpayers for Common Sense, <www.taxpayer.net/tcs/wastebasket/budget/3-16-01/pork.htm>.

5. Charles Lewis, *The Buying of Congress* (Washington, D.C.: Center for Public Integrity, 1998).

6. U.S. Bureau of the Census 2000, *Statistical Abstract of the United States, Table 549, Individual Income Tax Returns,* <www.census.gov/prod/2001pubs/statab.pdf>.

7. At the upper end of the benefits scale, the benefit is only 24 percent of what it is at the lower end per dollar of contributions. Additionally, higher-income retirees are taxed on 85 percent of their Social Security Benefit, perhaps at the highest rate of 37 percent.

8. U.S. Bureau of the Census 2000, *Statistical Abstract of the United States, Table 624, Supplementary Security Income* <www.census.gov/prod/2001pubs/statab.pdf>.

9. "Food stamp program participants and costs" U.S. Department of Agriculture Food and Nutrition Service, <www.fns.usda/pd/ssummar.htm>.

10. U.S. Bureau of the Census 2000, *Statistical Abstract of the United States, Table 538, Federal Outlays by Detailed Function,* <www.census.gov/prod/2001pubs/statab.pdf>.

11. U.S. Bureau of the Census 2000, *Statistical Abstract of the United States,* 2000, *Table 549, Individual Income Tax Returns,* <www.census.gov/prod/2001pubs/statab.pdf>.

12. Author's letter to the editors of *The Washington Post*, July 2, 1986. I stated the letter was not intended for publication, but included four pages of analysis and statistical tables. I presumed, rather naively, that the editors would at least admit the error.

15. *Factions*

1. For example, *see* Elizabeth Drew, *The Corruption of American Politics: What Went Wrong and Why* (New York: Overlook Press, 2000), especially pp. 61–85 (which cites Charles Lewis' *The Buying of Congress*).

16. *Professionalism*

1. Plutarch, *The Lives of the Noble Grecians and Romans, Great Books of the Western World*, volume 13 (Chicago: Encyclopedia Britannica, 1992), p. 649.

2. For example, see George Lundberg with George Stacey, *Severed Trust: Why American Medicine Hasn't Been Fixed* (New York: Basic Books, 2001). Dr. Lundberg, who was the editor of the *Journal of the American Medical Association* for seventeen years, strongly emphasizes the factor of greed.

3. "Ten questions for Ralph Nader," *Time*, August 5, 2002, p. 6.

Index

— U —

— V —

— W —

— Y —